D1454245

# A history of British sports medicine

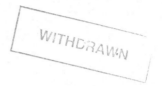

WITHDRAWN

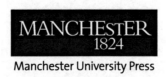

MANCHESTER
1824

Manchester University Press

HAMMERSMITH WEST LONDON COLLEGE

332685

# A history of British sports medicine

VANESSA HEGGIE

Manchester
University Press
Manchester and New York

distributed in the United States exclusively
by PALGRAVE MACMILLAN

Copyright © Vanessa Heggie 2011

The right of Vanessa Heggie to be identified as the author of this work has been asserted by her in accordance with the Copyright, Designs and Patents Act 1988.

Published by Manchester University Press
Oxford Road, Manchester M13 9NR, UK
and Room 400, 175 Fifth Avenue, New York, NY 10010, USA
www.manchesteruniversitypress.co.uk

Distributed in the United States exclusively by
Palgrave Macmillan, 175 Fifth Avenue,
New York, NY 10010, USA

Distributed in Canada exclusively by
UBC Press, University of British Columbia, 2029 West Mall,
Vancouver, BC, Canada V6T 1Z2

British Library Cataloguing-in-Publication Data is available

Library of Congress Cataloging-in-Publication Data is available

ISBN 978 0 7190 9128 5 paperback

First published by Manchester University Press in hardback 2011

This paperback edition first published 2013

The publisher has no responsibility for the persistence or accuracy of URLs for any external or third-party internet websites referred to in this book, and does not guarantee that any content on such websites is, or will remain, accurate or appropriate.

Printed by Lightning Source

HAMMERSMITH AND WEST
LONDON COLLEGE
LEARNING CENTRE

2 8 FEB 2014

332685   £14-99
617.1027 HEG
Sport
3WK

THE LEARNING CENTRE
HAMMERSMITH AND WEST
LONDON COLLEGE
GLIDDON ROAD
LONDON W14 9BL

# Contents

Acknowledgements                                          page vi
List of figures and boxes                                    viii
Abbreviations                                                   x

1   Introduction                                               1
2   Moderate individuals: beginnings, 1900–27                 25
3   Ideal citizens? Research and injuries, 1928–52            65
4   Making champions: boundaries, 1953–70                    104
5   Sport for All and the inert majority, 1970–87            145
6   Conclusion: specialty, 1988–2005                         183

Bibliography                                                 198
    Printed sources                                          198
    Government reports and resolutions                       214
    Websites                                                 214
    Archives                                                 216
Index                                                        219

# Acknowledgements

Much of the research for this book was carried out while I was working at the Centre for the History of Science, Technology and Medicine, University of Manchester, as a Research Associate on a three-year Wellcome Trust-sponsored project considering the history of sports medicine in the UK. I would like to thank the other project participants, particularly Ian Burney and Neil Carter for their help and advice. Subsequent research and writing was facilitated by a Mellon Post-doctoral Teaching Fellowship at the Department of History and Philosophy of Science, University of Cambridge. Three heads of department have helped steer my work – Mick Worboys, John Forrester and the much missed Peter Lipton. For invaluable advice on publishing, I'd also like to thank Jim Secord and Simon Schaffer. Neil Pemberton, Duncan Wilson, Rob Kirk and Nicky Reeves also contributed substantially to maintaining my sanity and improving my work. Many archivists and librarians have helped write this book, knowingly and unknowingly, and I'd like to specifically thank Amy Terriere at the British Olympic Association, and Natalie Milne of the then National Centre for Athletics Literature (now the Centre for Sports Science and History) at Birmingham University, for their friendly assistance. Dr Malcolm Read, Dr John Lloyd Parry MBE and Dr Robin Harland OBE have also offered support, information, and crucial practitioner insight, and I thank them all. All errors and opinions remain my own.

This book is dedicated to my parents, and to Ben, despite the fact that he thinks 6 am is a civilised time get up and go rowing.

# List of figures and boxes

*Figures*

page

1  The Olympic Village Hospital Los Angeles, 1932 and the Sports
   Medicine Centre at Montreal, 2007. [Upper image reproduced
   from the Official Report of the Xth Olympiad (p. 188) with the
   permission of the International Olympic Committee and
   remains © the IOC. Lower image © the author, 2007.]    13

2  Various treatments being delivered at the 'Footballers' Hospital',
   Matlock House in Manchester, c. 1899. [Efforts to trace the
   rights-holder were unsuccessful. Images reproduced with the
   permission of the Syndics of Cambridge University Library.]    27

3  A lesson in 'Anatomy' at Loughborough College, c. 1937. I would
   like to thank Jenny Clark, University Archivist at Loughborough
   University Library for her help tracing and identifying this
   image, which was used in promotional brochures. The brochure
   can also be found in the National Archives: NA ED113/3.    69

4  Athletes undergoing treatment at the Sports Injury Centre at
   the Crystal Palace National Sports Centre, c. 1990. [Reproduced
   from R Macdonald, 'Crystal Palace National Sports Centre –
   London, UK', BJSM 24 (1990), 10–12, with permission from
   BMJ Publishing Group Ltd.]    161

5  Opening Ceremony, Athens Olympic Games, 2004. [© Dr John
   Lloyd Parry, 2004. I extend my thanks to John for allowing me to
   reproduce this photograph.]    186

## Boxes

| | | page |
|---|---|---|
| 1 | The Footballers' Hospital | 61 |
| 2 | Adolphe Abrahams (1883–1967) | 62 |
| 3 | Staleness | 63 |
| 4 | Archibald Vivian Hill (1886–1977) | 101 |
| 5 | Arthur Espie Porritt (1900–94) | 102 |
| 6 | The Central Council of Physical Recreation (CCPR) | 103 |
| 7 | The Olympic medical archive (OMA) | 142 |
| 8 | Dr Lewis Griffiths Cresswell Evans Pugh (1909–94) | 143 |
| 9 | John GP Williams (1932–95) | 144 |
| 10 | Sports injuries clinics | 182 |

# Abbreviations

| | |
|---|---|
| AAA | Amateur Athletics Association |
| ACSM | American College of Sports Medicine |
| AIMS | Association Internationale Medico-Sportive |
| BAS(E)M | British Association of Sport and (Exercise) Medicine |
| BATS | British Association of Trauma in Sports |
| BBBC | British Boxing Board of Control |
| BJSM | British Journal of Sports Medicine |
| BMJ | British Medical Journal |
| BOA | British Olympic Association |
| CCPR | Central Council of Physical Recreation |
| DHSS | Department of Health and Social Security |
| FIMS | Fédération Internationale de Médecine Sportive |
| GLC | Greater London Council |
| IOC | International Olympic Committee |
| ISM | Institute of Sports Medicine (UK) |
| LSMI | London Sports Medicine Institute |
| MO | Medical Officer |
| MP | Member of Parliament |
| MRC | Medical Research Council |
| NASM | Netherlands Association of Sports Medicine |
| NFC | National Fitness Council |
| OMA | Olympic Medical Archives |
| RAMC | Royal Army Medical Corps |
| RCP | Royal College of Physicians |
| SIC | Sports Injuries Clinic |

# 1

# Introduction

In early December 1980, a 69-year-old woman was shot in the car park of an Ohio department store. She later died in hospital from her injuries, and initially her story was a sad but familiar one about an innocent bystander caught up in an armed robbery. But the results of an autopsy performed on her body caught media attention across the world, and even provoked representatives of international sports organisations to make official statements about her life and death.

Polish-born Stanisława Walasiewiczówna, better known by her Anglicised name, Stella Walsh, was a successful Olympian, with both a gold and silver medals in the 100m. She had been Polish sportsperson of the year for several years in the early 1930s, and had emigrated to the USA in 1947 when she married the boxer Neil Olsen. Although Walsh retired from competitive sports in 1951, she remained active in community and charity groups working with young athletes. The circumstances of her death in 1980 threatened to overshadow all these achievements when her autopsy revealed what are often coyly referred to as 'ambiguous' sexual features, or, as a member of the International Olympic Committee's Medical Commission put it, revealed that she 'was not a normal athlete from the femininity standpoint'.[1]

Walsh's death occurred at a moment when cheating was a particularly hot topic in sport, especially Olympic sport. The politically controversial summer Olympics in Moscow had just taken place, and the discussion of sexually ambiguous female competitors from the USSR and Eastern Europe went hand-in-hand with accusations of doping and steroid abuse.[2] The sudden revelation of a Polish gender fraud, her years living in the USA sometimes conveniently forgotten, fitted neatly into the storylines of sports journalists and other commentators. Despite pressure, the International Olympic Committee (IOC) decided not to rescind Walsh's medals, or remove her name from its record books. They argued that she had taken part in her events believing she was a woman, that the rules of the day would not necessarily have disqualified her, and that, essentially,

[w]hat happened almost half a century ago cannot be taken into account since there was no desire to break the regulations which were valid at the time, or indeed any awareness of having done so.[3]

Walsh's story takes us to the core of sports medicine in the twentieth century; its fundamental question, as this book will show, has been one of defining normality for the athlete. But Walsh's story is also a hint at the extraordinary mutability of sports medicine, where even something as apparently fundamental as biological gender could be redefined, re-codified, and reinterpreted over half a century. Just as the IOC recognised it would be anachronistic to take their existing definition of femininity and extend it retrospectively, so I have recognised, as far as possible, the pitfalls of making too many assumptions about what sports medicine 'should' look like in the past.

This is therefore a book in broad sympathy with other accounts of the social construction of disease and health.[4] As the section below will show, when interrogated, sports medicine is revealed as a complex, contingent and heterogeneous set of practices, beliefs and practitioners. Its appearance in the twenty-first century as a coherent object is the consequence of a set of interlaced scientific and social developments, and it is its construction as an object of special interest and expertise that is traced in this book. In a sentence, I argue that it is only when the athlete becomes 'not normal' – that is, both supernormal as well as abnormal – that one can have sports medicine as a distinct area of expertise. While the athlete remains normal, and by implication healthy, what we have is medicine applied to sport. This book describes how and why, in Britain, medicine applied to sport became first an area of expertise known as sports medicine, and then a formal medical specialty: Sport and Exercise Medicine.

### What is sports medicine?

Histories of disciplines or professions always risk becoming teleological. In seeking origins it is easy to develop a sense of inevitability about the development of some activities, while anything that is not part of modern practice can be judged as ill-conceived, a detour away from the 'real story' and simply irrelevant. Sports medicine was recognised as a formal specialty in the UK in 2005, and gained its first British organisation – the British Association of Sport and (Exercise) Medicine (BAS(E)M) – in 1952.[5] A narrowly conceived history could wind between these two events, seeing little that it is willing to acknowledge as 'sports medicine' prior to the 1930s or 1940s when the founders of BAS(E)M began to show their interest in sports and exercise physiology. Such a history would probably recapitulate the assertion that twentieth-century British sports medicine was backwards on the world stage and retarded by an ingrained spirit of voluntary and non-professional practice.[6]

It would also be an incomplete history. By 1900 there was an institution known as the 'Footballers' Hospital' established in Manchester and treating foreign as well as British athletes; by the early twentieth century nearly every training manual for sports claimed to be scientifically informed or to be using the latest medical understandings of the body; in 1908 the first rules against doping were introduced by the hosts at the London-based Olympic Games; in the 1920s a Briton won a Nobel Prize for his early work on lactic acid metabolism and went on to do pioneering research in exercise physiology; by the 1930s several sporting organisations were engaging (although sometimes on a voluntary basis) medical professionals of all kinds to support their members; when the NHS was founded in 1948 it contained at least one clinic specialising in the care of injured athletes. To be sufficient, a history of sports medicine in Britain needs to contextualise these facts.

Of course, there is the opposite problem where, by seeking the origins of a current practice in the ambiguity of the past, nearly everything seems to be relevant. This is made a more serious complication by the nature of sports medicine itself; modern specialists identify it as a highly diverse, multi-practitioner, multi-disciplinary, multi-specialty activity.[7] By the 1960s, even if we take the narrowest view of sports medicine and limit it to just the members of BAS(E)M, this could still include general practitioners, a range of different consultant and specialist surgeons, gynaecologists, paediatricians, dieticians, physiotherapists, masseurs, physiologists, exercise scientists, psychologists, members of the armed forces, teachers of physical education, coaches and trainers, volunteers for organisations like St John Ambulance, and medical students. Practice is as diverse; the range from first-aid on the pitch to highly specialised surgical and medical intervention is obvious, but it is not as clear where this should include sports science research, or the use of exercise as a therapy.

As if this was not enough, sports medicine and its constituents are highly unstable categories; biomedical ideas about what was normal and healthy for the athlete, or what role medicine could and should play in sport, vary considerably between 1905 and 2005. So what this book will do is avoid some teleology, some confusion, by not trying to tell a story about a consistent idea but by emphasising instead sports medicine's inconsistency (its different constructions). The dramatic way in which the very *idea* of sports medicine has changed over a century is the core of this text. The question, 'what is normal for the athlete?', has changed significantly; at the beginning of the twentieth century the definition of the normal athlete essentially overlapped with that of the normal, healthy citizen. Through the years that followed, these categories were gradually separated, as the athletic body began to be medically, scientifically and socially constructed as a discrete physiological or clinical entity.

It was this distinction between normal athlete and normal citizen that allowed sports medicine to identify itself as a medical specialism by the 1950s and consolidate this position in the 1960s. In the later decades of the twentieth century this definition became problematic not only for sports medicine, but also for politicians, civil servants and sports organisations. The 'leisure revolution' and concurrent attempts by government to include sport and exercise more prominently in public health measures has required a new understanding of the relationship between the athlete and the normal citizen. Sports doctors and sports scientists have had to find ways to map their specialist knowledge of the athlete back onto the body public. That this is not always successful (or desirable) can be illustrated by the struggles emerging from the London 2012 programme; while 'legacy' is a regularly repeated buzzword, what an Olympic athlete demands from, say, a swimming pool, is quite different to the needs of a local community with a population of young and old, able-bodied and disabled.[8] Likewise, an emphasis on exercise for health has a complicated relationship with the increasing biomedical evidence that elite athletes are neither healthy nor long-lived.

Sports medicine is a practice that has been defined by the nature of its patients. Unlike other specialties, which focus on regions of the body, disease types, specific body tissues, or techniques and technological interventions, sports medicine does as paediatrics and geriatrics do, and claims expertise in a particular 'sort' of human being. Unlike paediatrics and geriatrics, however, it is not a life-stage, but an activity which initially defines the patient group; to become a specialty there had to be evidence that this activity actually created abnormal human types, which needed specialist handling. Thus the construction of sports medicine has been affected by both scientific and social changes, which this book will describe by focusing on biomedical understandings of the athletic body: what is an athlete, who treats them, and why?

Asking these questions about the patient, about the athletic body, makes sense of the diversity and mutability of sports medicine over the twentieth century. It also ensures that we are able to transcend the expectation that sports medicine in 1905 always ought to resemble, or at least lead to, the formal specialty of 2005. At the least, athletes have had the same access to health care as any of their peers; therefore, when a patient gains different or specialised treatment or advice, either because he or she is an athlete or because he or she is taking part in sport, we can begin to see a divide between sports medicine and other, related, branches of biomedicine and health care.

### What does sports medicine do? Cure, prevention and enhancement

Like most other forms of medicine, sports medicine is interested in both the prevention and the cure of disease, sickness and injury. 'Prevention' in sports medicine often involves a high level of medical policing, from emphasising suitable warm-up exercises and stretches through to instituting weight categories and mandating the use of protective clothing during competition. As in other specialties, cure can be immediate or long-term, including rehabilitation and the retraining of injured bodies. But what makes sports medicine stand out is that it has a third area of interest: enhancing the human body. Unlike every other branch of medical practice, with the possible exception of some areas of plastic surgery, it is not solely concerned with returning unhealthy, abnormal bodies to their usual, normal, or healthy state, much less to making bodies 'average'. Instead, it is also interested in the enhancement of a normal body so that it can perform extraordinary, often intrinsically dangerous, feats of physical achievement and endurance.

Because of this interest, sports medicine can sometimes invert normal medical ethics. A sports doctor may be asked to care for a patient for the express purpose of allowing them to inflict physical harm on another human being; or, more often, to inflict physical harm on themselves through high-impact sports and high-intensity, unsustainable training regimes. They may be asked to prioritise a short-term goal, a sporting ambition, over long-term health risks (such as early-onset arthritis). It is this strange feature – enhancement – which has so far attracted most scholarly attention, at the expense of discussions of the many other features of sports medicine.

But the boundaries between these fields are porous, and practices which in one decade are enhancement could in others be more legitimately seen as treatment or prevention. The clearest example is training; training can be conceptualised as a form of enhancement, taking a normal body and enlarging, expanding, even redesigning it for the purposes of sport. And yet it is quite clear that for many training manuals prior to the 1910s the purpose of training was, rather, to regain lost health, to create a perfectly 'normal' body for sport. If anything, such texts are preventive medicine, ensuring that the sedentary office worker is in a fit state to take part in sport beneficially, and showing him/her pictures of appropriate technique so that he/she does not strain or sprain a muscle or tendon. (A similar argument about a transition from cure/prevention to enhancement has recently been made by Beamish and Ritchie in relation to the use of ergogenic substances and drugs.)[9]

## Dope, drugs and cheating

There is a rich sociological as well as historical literature on the ethics and practice of doping and enhancement, much of which supports the arguments made in this book.[10] The number of studies of enhancement (particularly doping and drug testing) compared to the thin literature on any other areas of sports medicine, demonstrates our fascination with this unique aspect of sports medicine; but this book will show that considering sports medicine as a multi-faceted practice adds depth and context to some of the conclusions of such work. For example, John Hoberman's *Mortal Engines* concentrates specifically on enhancement, mostly doping and psychological techniques, and with a particular emphasis on communist and fascist sports science in the twentieth century. Nonetheless, many of the themes of his work are echoed in the broader history of sports medicine outlined here. In particular, he identifies a shift from an 'older doctrine of natural limits [to a] new doctrine of expanding biological limits' around 1900, the changing 'ontology of human performance' noted by Beamish and Ritchie (although they locate it later in the century, around 1930), which I discuss in Chapter 2.[11] Similarly, the connections Hoberman notes between the military and athletic body are also of relevance here, in Chapter 3, and the ongoing desire to delineate between normal/abnormal and physiological/pathological is a theme throughout *Mortal Engines* and this book.

As well as enriching the current literature on enhancement, this account of the history of the athletic body also offers new lines of explanation. Some histories of sports have considered the appearance of drug testing in the middle of the twentieth century as a symptom of corrupted sports, often claiming that professionalism and commercialisation have driven athletes to extremes for the rewards of winning.[12] More recent sports studies scholarship tends instead to argue that athletes have always taken drugs, and that they have always looked to ergogenic substances to help them train and win. Further, sports sociologists and bioethicists have problematised notions of drug definitions and 'cheating', querying the artificial and often arbitrary boundaries between acceptable and unacceptable chemicals and doses.[13] It is no longer tenable to explain the development of extensive and costly drug testing procedures in the middle of the twentieth century as a simple moral reaction against increased 'cheating' in sport.

Hoberman instead points to a longer history of enhancement, where the body is a complicated amalgam of racial and national identity, and where sport and sporting ethics can become shorthand for political and social ideologies. Much of the drug crisis, he suggests, is a phenomenon of the Cold War, of the 'us and them' mentality present in international sport. More recent scholarship offers other analyses: for Paul Dimeo, drug testing in sport reflects drug use in society; a prevailing European Christian social morality and a middle-class Anglo-Saxon attitude to sports imposed an anti-drug rhetoric on international sport, which was entirely unreflective of the longer history of athletic enhancement or of contemporary sporting practice.[14] This book offers a third interpretation; it is only by describing athletic bodies as different to normal bodies that enhancement, particularly by drugs, becomes an area of negotiation for new rules and new biomedical categories of control.

At the beginning of the twentieth century the athletic body was considered to be an exemplar of healthy normality. Under this understanding, athletes took a range of drugs and ergogenic aids (from cocoa to cocaine) as legitimate medicinal substances to help alleviate pain or fatigue. Obviously, as social attitudes shifted some of these substances became associated with danger or addiction or immoral practice, but the principle – that if it's morally acceptable for the banker then it's morally acceptable for the high jumper – remained the same. But when athletes became something else, super- or sub-normal, heroes or avatars, they were subject to different rules. As their bodies were described as distinct clinical entities, with their own special needs and specialist medical practitioners, they also began to be regulated much more tightly than 'normal' people; now substances like caffeine, alcohol, even oxygen, could be considered problematic.

Changing attitudes towards drug taking and pharmaceuticals in general may have played a role in the demonisation of doping, but what is special about sport now is the high standard of purity it requires, a fundamental change over the twentieth century. In the 1930s the use of gland extracts in professional Association Football was controversial (see Chapter 3), but for many of the same reasons it might be so when used to invigorate the tired city worker.[15] There was no suggestion at this time that the footballer taking glands for personal, medical, reasons should be excluded from competition. In the early twenty-first century it looks likely that the impotent male athlete will have to choose between erectile dysfunction and a suspension for the use of Viagra during competition.[16] Other sufferers in other walks of life do not have international authorities demanding that they choose between losing their jobs and putting up with sexual dysfunction; different bodies, different rules. In addition, drug testing requires the presence of experts to conduct and design the tests, to research the use of drugs, to enforce the bans, to educate athletes – all of this infrastructure comes with the development of mainstream sports medicine. The apparently sudden concern with the purity of athletic bodies in the mid-twentieth century is certainly partly an effect of the Cold War, as well as being a feature of changing social and cultural attitudes towards drug taking. But it was also part of broader developments in sports medicine.

The recent history of enhancement reveals an 'untold story' which will be added to in this book – that British scientists, doctors and athletes played a central role in the development of dope tests and doping regulations.[17] The centrality of Britain, and the world-leading nature of British sports medicine may come as a surprise, because it is common to hear British sports medicine described by practitioners (at all points in the twentieth century) as backwards on the world stage; underfunded, undervalued and unprofessional.[18] On occasions, this attitude has been reinforced by historians; instead, Germany is described as the primary nation in terms of the development of enhancement processes and state-organised sport, or the USA is centralised because of its highly commercialised and professionalised attitude towards sports from high-school to the Olympic level.

### Amateurism and history: sport and medicine

So despite John Welshman's 1998 plea that the history of medicine and sports history should 'only connect', and despite the publications on drugs, doping and enhancement, general British sports medicine has so far attracted little historical interest.[19] There is a potted (and extra-national) history: perhaps passing reference is made to Hippocrates' ambiguous attitude towards the Greek athlete, or of Galen's practice on the gladiators of the *circus maximus*. Then many centuries are skipped to often lurid accounts of boxers' or professional walkers' ('pedestrians') diet and training in the early 1800s before some developments in exercise physiology at the end of the nineteenth century are discussed. These seem to lead naturally to institutional and academic developments in Germany in the 1920s. Then in 1928 the first international sports medicine organisation is formed, followed only in the 1950s by BAS(E)M, and then the story moves to further institutions, to drug and gender testing, to commercialisation and televisation. If there is any conclusion, it is the rather uninformative one that sport was somehow 'medicalised' over the twentieth century, usually as a result of commercial and economic pressures.[20] So far the complexity of this process of 'medicalisation' has largely remained unexplored. Partly this is because interest has focused on the social history of sport and medicine, where physical education and physical culture have proved more interesting than the sort of sports medicine outlined here, and have been particularly well explored in terms of gender and identity history.[21] In the only edited volume directly relating to sports medicine, Berryman and Park's *Sport and Exercise Science: Essays in the History of Sports Medicine*, just two of the ten chapters consider sports medicine after 1920, and half focus on North America or Germany alone – none on Britain alone.[22]

Probably the most prolific writer on sports medicine, Roberta Park, has concentrated on the period around 1900, and generally discusses Britain only in close connection with developments in the USA.[23] She and others have tended to present a picture of Victorian and Edwardian Britain populated by sceptical doctors who apparently took very cautionary stances on the value of exercise and regularly warned of its potential dangers.[24] Here, in Chapter 2, and elsewhere I have shown that there are other interpretations of the materials used in these studies; I believe that the British medical and scientific professions had a much more robust take on exercise and fatigue, with most mainstream textbooks downplaying the risks of even the most vigorous exercise on the bodies of young, fit, men.[25] (The potential effects on those who were not young adults, male or healthy, were certainly more ambiguous).

Later in the century this sceptical role is allegedly taken up by sports administrators, coaches and athletes themselves. According to some accounts, the fears of doctors around 1900 led them to attempt to repress, restrict or control sporting achievement, and in return sportsmen 'resisted' medical control, leading to a lack of development in British sports science and the delayed formation of formal sports medicine organisations.[26] As this book will show, such an argument is unsupported by the evidence. In Britain, by the late nineteenth century, writings on sport and medicine show no consensus that vigorous exercise was unhealthy per se, and although Britain was rarely world-leading in the sophistication of its institutions or the significance of its research, it has hardly been the lagging nation in terms of the provision of health care to athletes, development of sports medicine organisations, or even the recognition of sports medicine as a specialty.

Why should such a myth about British sports medicine endure? Firstly because sports history and the history of medicine are distinct disciplines, and interdisciplinary work between these fields is relatively rare.[27] Without an adequate understanding of the average person's access to health care in the 1930s, the extensive and extraordinary provision of masseurs, UV-lamp therapy and faradic baths to footballers may seem archaic. It is easy to laugh at photographs of Olympic sprinters smoking shortly before or after competing, but this is not an indication of an 'amateur attitude' in the 1940s or 1950s where the connections between lung health and smoking were not as unambiguous as they are today.

The second reason is amateurism itself, the tensions and contradictions of which fill several volumes.[28] It is difficult to overstate how important the notion of amateurism is to the history of British sport (or, at least, to *historians* of British sport). It is a widely used explanatory factor for attitudes in and towards sport, and for developments in British and colonial sporting practice. Yet definitions of amateurism are slippery and hard to come by. In its most simplistic formula, the amateur/professional divide is merely one of finance, where the professional is paid to take part in sport and the amateur is not. Of course, even this definition has many interpretations – are board and lodgings 'payment'? Or compensation for lost wages?

Amateurism is also an attitude, one claimed as intrinsic by many nations and generations, and open to wide reinterpretation. It is often depicted as a particularly British trait, emerging from the great Victorian public schools and their sporting ethos; this interpretation centralises the gentleman-amateur who plays for the love of the game, not for financial reward or even the desire to win. Here is the origin of many of the familiar phrases about sport, where things are 'fair game' or 'not cricket'. Of course, as recent critiques of the use of 'amateurism' as an explanatory force have pointed out, there is not one but many kinds of amateurism, redefined according to class, gender, nationality, and varying between sports, between nations and over time. It is a highly mutable ideology that can be mobilised to justify a wide range of socio-political attitudes towards sport and the correct conduct of sporting events.

To take an example specifically relevant to sports medicine; in the 1960s there was a great deal of debate about the ethics of holding the 1968 Olympic Games in Mexico City, at mid-altitude. It was believed that this height would affect unacclimatised athletes and their performances, while advantaging the few sportspeople who happened to have been born or live at mid-altitude. Amateurism as a creed offered no clear answer to this problem, while all those involved in the debate claimed that *they* were the ones protecting the great amateur spirit of the Olympics. Perhaps the true amateur competed for the love of the game, and so just accepted any environmental disadvantages, as he/she was there to enjoy the sport rather than just to win. On the other hand, perhaps the defenders of amateurism should fight against a venue which would unfairly advantage those who could afford expensive altitude training (see Chapter 4).[29]

'Amateur' can also be a critical epithet, particularly in the case of sports medicine. Amateurism in attitude would surely retard the take-up of technical and scientific interventions, while amateurism in practice meant the persistence of a voluntary tradition in sports, where professionals were not paid for their services. But this neglects the fact that amateurism could easily be mobilised to support highly technical activities – dope testing, for example, is regularly referred to as a form of defence against over-competitive athletes who are not properly imbued with the 'spirit of amateurism'. Arguing that amateurism tends to retard the use of technical skills also ignores the fact that professional service given voluntarily is still *professional*. Medicine in particular has a strong voluntary tradition; the unpaid work by doctors and surgeons for athletes and sportspeople mirrors in interesting ways the unpaid work of consultants in the Victorian voluntary hospitals, who gained status from their (unpaid) hospital positions while earning an income from private patients.[30]

This is not to suggest that casual hiring practices (or the failure of team managers to secure consistent and regular medical care) had no effect on sports medicine. Certainly by the 1970s sports medicine practitioners and sporting bodies were vocally criticising the failings of some sports organisations, and many sought a more formalised and regulated provision of sports medicine to athletes at all levels. Yet to call all these practitioners 'amateurs' simply because they were not paid for the hours they spent with the Olympic team or football club is misleading. Volunteers, certainly, but to assume that the financial definition of amateurism necessarily goes hand-in-hand with unprofessional practice is, in this case, an error.

The flexibility of the term 'amateurism' means that it is not possible meaningfully to sum up the influence of British amateurism (if any such beast exists) on the development of sports medicine, any more than it is possible to sum up the influence of medicine on the development of British sport merely by using the word 'medicalised'. Amateurism is itself so contingent on specific sporting traditions, and on the socio-cultural work it is supposed to be doing in any scenario, that its effect cannot be conclusively identified and is probably secondary to the many other influences – local club culture, legal frameworks, political ambitions – which themselves alter the meaning and function of sporting amateurism.

In a very basic form, the financial consequences of the amateur/ professional divide in British sport have necessarily had some effect on the way sports medicine is practised. When a profit is being made from sport there is obviously going to be money which could be invested in medical care, insurance or research. But if we compare the two largest professional sports in Britain, Association Football and boxing, we see they have had different patterns of medical provision; so that the development of a professional and an amateur sport (boxing) may be more closely related than two professional sports (boxing and football). Professional boxing formalised its medical services in the first half of the twentieth century, introducing a Chief Medical Officer in 1946 and a full Medical Committee under the Boxing Board of Control in 1950.[31] It seems that this was done at least in part to deflect increasing criticisms from the medical profession about the possible dangers of boxing – criticisms specific to this sport, and shared by amateur as well as professional boxing (amateur boxing had also established medical surveillance of bouts by the 1940s). Association Football has had, if anything, even more extensive provision. After a court case in 1912, footballers were legally considered manual workers, and were therefore covered by the 1911 National Insurance Act. But, as Chapter 3 shows, provision was often above and beyond these legal requirements, as footballers often had access to healthcare facilities unavailable to either the amateur athlete or other manual labourers.[32] Yet those involved with British football seem to struggle with the apparent conflict between a rugged working-class ideology of sport and the use of high-technology science and medicine.[33] Rhetoric and reality need not match.

What this tells us is that we need a finer grained approach to the history of sport and medicine, of exercise and health. Catch-all explanations like 'amateurism' or 'medicalisation' do not actively explain what was happening in Britain in the twentieth century. Instead of a 'medicalisation' or 'amateurism' hypothesis, this book provides a history of sports medicine as an idea, and later as a practice and specialty in Britain, which, roughly speaking, should provide a good pattern for the development of sports medicine in other nations. It has its nationally specific features, and the rhetoric of amateurism is one, alongside the practical implications of nationalised healthcare provision. Additionally, British scientists, politicians, doctors and athletes were central figures in most major international sports and sports medicine organisations, and British research was part of an international common language of exercise physiology and sports science.

### The athletic body in context

My concentration on the athletic body has led to a focus on elite (national level and above) athletes, and consequently school sports, physical culture and exercise for health are marginalised in this story. This is not just my prejudice; it is clear that the first institutions of British sports medicine focused on the elite body at the expense of the schoolchild or casual sportsperson. It could have been possible for sports medicine to be constructed as a version of public health or healthy living, but that is not, in the end, what happened in Britain. (There is certainly a need for a history which laces together the excellent work done on physical culture in the first half of the twentieth century with material covering the second half, which seems to concentrate more on personal identity and body image).[34]

Government interest in sports and exercise, for the general public as

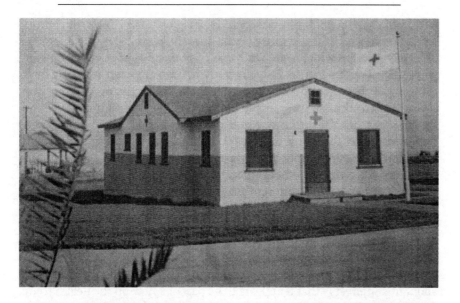

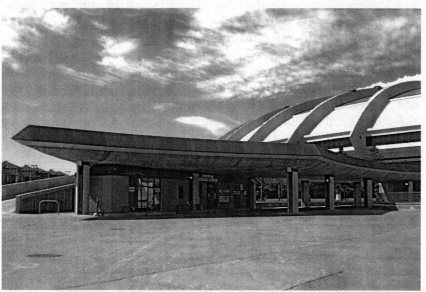

**1.** The Olympic Village Hospital Los Angeles, 1932 and the Sports Medicine Centre at Montreal, 2007. The first Olympic Village was built in 1932 at the Los Angeles Olympiad, and it contained the first Olympic Hospital. By the end of the twentieth century the idea of 'legacy' for the Olympic Games means that many facilities remain in place for the use of the non-Olympic sportsman and woman after the Games. The lower picture shows the sports medicine centre at Montreal's Olympic Stadium Park (2007).

well as the schoolchild, has waxed and waned over the twentieth century. At the beginning of the century it was only the physical exercise regimes of 'captive' bodies which were really the responsibility of government, and while school sports (particularly for women) have attracted scholarly inter-est, comparably extensive work on exercise in the army, or in the prison, asylum and workhouse remains to be done.[35] This interest broadened into the 'nation's health' in the war and inter-war periods, including diet as well as exercise; the irony, as this book will show, is that this interest in part contributed to the split between elite sports and lay sport, and in turn reinforced the claims by emerging sports medicine specialists in the 1940s that their patients were 'different'.

Although I do not specifically address the history of public health, recent work in that area has informed some of the arguments in this book. In particular, the re-emergence of government interest (and the interest of tax-funded, non-governmental bodies, such as the Sports Council) in sport and exercise in the 1970s is crucial to Chapter 5. What is significant about this interest is that it appears to be part of a new public health trend, described by Virginia Berridge and characterised by, firstly, concerns about diseases with a complicated association between risk and reward, which entailed the use of statistics and epidemiological studies; secondly, a tendency to use mass media, sometimes having doctors address the public directly; and thirdly, an emphasis on individual lifestyle and behav-iour.[36] All three of these characteristics can be seen in the interest and ten-sions surrounding the Sport for All movement, and debates over whether 'the government' should be seen to be encouraging sport and exercise for health. These issues are touched on in Chapter 5, but require closer examination in their own right.

Tracing the history of the athletic body also means that some sources which are useful in early chapters are relied on less heavily in later ones, and vice versa. For example, this work is not intended to provide a history of science and medicine in sports training and the training manual; train-ing manuals provide a vital source of information about the athletic body in the early twentieth century, before organisations, institutions, and specialist sports medicine texts begin to provide insights. Consequently they are used heavily in Chapter 2, and hardly at all by Chapter 5. Gaps in the archival records also impose limitations; few materials from the London Olympics in 1908 remain, while the records of the Sports Council for the early 1980s seem to have been lost. Oral histories have been used, although some of the difficulty of amateur rhetoric make it difficult to gain accounts of drug use (even when it was legal), or the adoption of 'scientific' training practices.[37]

Finally: the male pronoun predominates. Throughout the twentieth century the majority of practitioners of sports medicine, and the majority of their patients (at least, the patients they discussed) have been men. The gender of the athletic body has been, by default, male. There are fascinating stories to be told about women's participation in the construction of this body, and about its effect on female athletes and medical professionals, and those should have a book of their own. This text concentrates on mainstream sports medicine, which strongly and consistently gendered male; it is also adult, and usually white.

## Conclusions

The following chapters proceed in chronological fashion from the late nineteenth century to specialisation in 2005. While this is a history of sports medicine – prevention, treatment and enhancement – clearly it draws on developments in exercise physiology and sports science. The division between sports science and medicine is a porous one, although most historical actors seem to have experienced little difficulty in knowing where the line lay.[38] My focus on the body makes the division clearer – while sports scientists certainly experimented on the athletic body, that work still required the intervention of sports medicine to transform it into a practice of relevance to the athletic body as a patient. So while this book centralises medicine, some prominent sports scientists and some developments in exercise physiology are discussed. Likewise, although this book centres on Britain, Britain's place 'in the world' is not neglected. Research from across the globe affects British sports medicine, as did the rules of international sports organisations and, in the second half of the twentieth century, pressure from European organisations. Chapter 6 discusses sports medicine in other nations, and the rest of the book includes specific accounts of medical provision and scientific research at every summer Olympic Games from Athens in 1896 to Los Angeles in 1984. (The Olympics are also useful because of their periodicity, providing a snapshot of medical provision at relatively regular intervals).

Other historians have located the 'beginning' of sports medicine as early as the late nineteenth century, and as late as the 1920s, and Chapter 2 covers this problematic period. I make no argument that there is any sort of organised sports medicine in Britain at this point, nor that the activities of doctors or scientists working with athletes and in sports were anything but marginal. It is essential, however, to understanding why sports medical institutions were founded, and sports medicine textbooks were written, *after* this period by demonstrating why it did not happen earlier. Organised and regulated sporting activity was a significant feature of Victorian British culture; concerns about degenerate working-class populations, military strength and weakly urban children provoked a renewed interest in muscular Christianity, school exercise and physical 'hygiene' of all kinds.[39] It is a reasonable question to ask why a sports or exercise medicine tradition did not emerge in association with the new sports governing bodies, to treat those engaged in the crazes of tennis or of cycling, or to deal with the pressing issue of female sporting activity.[40]

Chapter 2 answers this question by demonstrating that in these early years the athletic body was still conceptualised as normal, and by default 'healthy'. Much sports medicine was therefore rather 'medicine applied to sport'. Vigorous exercise was an acceptable, probably necessary, part of the moderate healthy lifestyle for the normal, healthy man. Consequently sports medicine was part and parcel of normal medical treatment, distinguishable only through its location (on the field) or through its patient history (i.e. treating a sports-related injury). This is clearly demonstrated by attitudes towards dope and doping, where if drugs were condemned at all, it was because they might cause a healthy man to over-reach his natural limits. Even the most strident advocates of British amateurism recommended strychnine injections to 'pep-up' long distance runners, or a drink of brandy to stimulate fatigued footballers. Yet, importantly, in this time period sports medicine did for the first time find a distinctive niche, and that was in the support and surveillance of the bodies of those who were *not* healthy young men engaging in normal sporting events. Extraordinary events (like the marathon) required extraordinary medical consideration; hidden disease (particularly heart disease) needed to be rooted out by doctors before people could safely take part in sports; male children particularly needed guidance from medical professionals, as their bodies were not necessarily as fitted for exercise as the normal bodies of adult men. Women and girls had, of course, already been identified as abnormal by other medical professionals, and their exclusion from physical activity was part of a larger, non-sport-specific construction of their physiology.[41]

Chapter 2 also demonstrates that there was no wide-spread *de facto* scepticism about the value of vigorous exercise among physicians and scientists. It shows instead that concepts such as 'individualism' and 'moderation' could be used as organising principles in sports medicine. They could also be used by both athletes and scientists to judge the value of training schemes or evaluate statements about the health risks and benefits of training regimes and lifestyles. Chapter 2 also gives two specific examples of where the athletic body gained treatment systems that only later became mainstream; the use of exercise rather than rest for soft tissue and orthopaedic injuries, and the use of 'scientific' massage. Both these belie accounts which suggest that because of amateurism athletes resisted the inclusion of novelty or 'scientific' ideas in their training regimes.

The normality of the young male athlete was reconsidered between 1928 and 1952, the period covered by Chapter 3. At the beginning of this chapter the athlete is still a normal man, and an 'ideal citizen'. By the end he is something quite different, an abnormal or supernormal human being who demands and requires specialist medical interventions. There were three key factors which influenced this shift, mostly related to the changes in organisation and understanding of the biomedical sciences forced by two world wars. Firstly, wartime needs led to increased state interest in, and funding for, research and clinical specialisms relevant to sports medicine.[42] The soldier's body shares a great deal in common with the athletic body; both are unusual patient groups in that they are often male, usually fit and healthy (aside from traumatic or exercise injury), and are generally young. Those working on soldiers in wartime have found athletes to be a clear patient model in peacetime. Secondly, this interest extended to the civilian population through a perceived need to improve general fitness, as well as specific challenges such as maintaining a healthy population under the ration book. Physical culture systems from European nations – particularly, of course, Germany – were looked to with concern (and sometimes envy), resulting in the setting up of various institutions and organisations to consider the relationships between exercise and health, and increase public access to exercise facilities. Thirdly, sport became explicitly a site for international conflict. Demands for higher performances and better regulation led both professional and amateur sports to formalise their medical rules.

Consequently there emerged a body of doctors, physiologists and medical auxiliaries with experience in research relevant to sports, and sometimes specifically with experience in competition and with athletes. These interested and experienced professionals – coming from military research, civilian fitness schemes or sport itself – congregated on organisations' sub-committees, on governmental advisory groups and the like. Their advice was actively sought by athletes, trainers and coaches as the levels of performance in international sports improved (often leaving British sportsmen and women out of the running). These disparate individuals began to organise themselves and recognise themselves as a distinct group of medical specialists.

By the 1950s elite athletes were definitely different to the rest of us, and in Chapter 4 (1953–70) I discuss how specialist organisations dedicated to the study and treatment of this different body appeared in Britain. Once athletes were medically described as a clinically distinct patient group, it was possible to justify sports medicine as a specialism, an area of expertise at least, if not yet a formal specialty. Consequently the 1950s and 1960s were a period of boundary formation in Britain, which are reflective of developments in international sports medicine. Boundaries were being drawn around this new athletic body: because athletes were not normal, then what was 'normal for the athlete' needed to be defined. It is no coincidence that the major topics debated in sports medicine at this time were the introduction of at-event dope and gender testing, both issues clearly about what should to be considered normal and abnormal for the athlete.

Doctors already had the authority to dictate who could and who could not take part in sport through early screening activities applied to vulnerable bodies and extraordinary sports. By the 1960s this control had expanded to cover all elite athletes, and many others, who could be declared the wrong gender, too heavy or too light, or found to have taken a banned substance; such decisions could end careers and wreck lives. The organisations and institutions which sought some part of this control of the athletic body also struggled to maintain their own boundaries, and claim authority in this newly significant medical field. Chapter 4 discusses the formation and work of BAS(E)M, the Institute of Sports Medicine (ISM), the Sports Council, and the British Olympic Association's Medical Committee. All these organisations claimed intellectual and financial territory within sports medicine, and therefore power over the athletic body. These boundary disputes were sometimes extremely acrimonious, and continued for the rest of the century, as Chapters 5 and 6 will show.

Having justified their expertise by an appeal to the elite body, sports medicine practitioners found challenging the period from the 1970s. New political agendas (such as the Sport For All movement) began to increase governmental interest and intervention in sport and exercise; epidemiological research seemed to show that exercise and sport might be answers to the increasingly expensive diseases of civilisation – particularly heart disease (and here is a situation where training is not just preventive medicine and enhancement, but also becomes a form of treatment). Periods of increased prosperity, the leisure revolution, and the popularisation of exercise for health all introduced new patient bodies into the world of sports medicine. The specialism's successful reinterpretation of the athletic body (and thus its patient group) in the last quarter of the twentieth century, even changing the discipline's name to 'sport *and exercise* medicine', was vital to its survival.

Sports medicine faced two dangers; firstly that sports might be entirely normalised, so that sports medicine would be absorbed within other branches of everyday healthcare provision. This would be an unwelcome return to the situation before 1928, described in Chapter 2, so that the specialism of Chapter 4 became a passing phase before sports medicine merged back into generalised public health, school sports, etc. Secondly, elite sport was increasingly being abstracted from mass participation sport and exercise for fitness – with different government departments, funding streams and so on. Clinging to this elite, abnormal patient body would result in a tiny patient pool, limiting sport medicine's growth as a profession (and probably excluding it from the interest of the NHS). Instead, as Chapter 5 describes, a new construction of sports medicine successfully absorbed the lay sporting body into its articulations of the elite sporting body. Sport was figured rhetorically as a drug, something which was given out 'on prescription' and which required medical surveillance – for healthy 'normal' bodies and those 'at risk' alike.

At the same time, the organisations and institutions of sports medicine founded in the 1950s and 1960s began to formally shore up the boundaries of their specialism, to secure the definition of sports medicine into the future. What had been an area of expertise based on experience, networks and tacit knowledge was gradually replaced by a formalised medical specialism with courses, diplomas and certificates, eventually becoming a formal medical specialty. Chapter 6 completes the story of this development from 1987 to 2005, and then compares the pace and chronology of specialty formation in the UK to countries worldwide. In many cases British sports medicine was formalised and institutionalised before other countries, *pace* the regular critiques within Britain (sometimes by historians) of British sports medicine as 'backwards' on the world stage. Perhaps most notable is the fact that, despite any romantic notions about British amateurism, Britain was only the second country, after Germany, to base its sports medicine around the elite athletic body rather than instituting it as a sideline to general fitness and public health interests.

Chapter 6 also abstracts the process of specialisation in sports medicine and compares it to other accounts of medical and scientific specialisation. Then the chapter turns to fitness. The athlete has often been used to represent 'fitness', but a more important question to ask is, surely, 'fit for what?'.[43] The answer to that question – normal life, war, elite competition – gives us an insight into how athletic bodies are conceptualised, and how sports medicine has formed and reformed over a century. Normal, supernormal and abnormal, it is by understanding the athletic body that we can understand sports medicine.

One final note: because so little has been written on sports medicine to date, this book should also serve as a starting point for the fine-grained research that this topic needs. Partly to facilitate that, some areas of interest, some biographies, key words, and so on, have been discussed separately to the main text, in boxes which can be found at the end of each chapter.

## Notes

1 E Hay, 'The Stella Walsh Case' *Olympic Review* 162 (1981), 221–2. 222. For more on Walsh and gender testing, see Chapter 4.

2 J Hoberman, *Mortal Engines: The Science of Performance and the Dehumanization of Sport*, (New Jersey: Blackburn Press, 1992), particularly Chapter 4 'Faster, Higher, Stronger: A History of Doping in Sport', pp. 100–53 and Chapter 6 'The Myth of Communist Sports Science', pp. 193–228.

3 Hay, 'The Stella Walsh Case', 222.

4 This is a literature too large to cite comprehensively. Starting points are L Jordanova, 'The Social Construction of Medical Knowledge', *Social History of Medicine* 8 (1995), 361–81 and more generally J Golinski, *Making Natural Knowledge: Constructivism and the History of Science* (Chicago; London: University of Chicago Press, 2005).

5 The British Association of Sport and Medicine added 'and Exercise' to its name in 1999; it is often wrongly referred to as the British Association of Sports Medicine.

6 As an example, see M Cronin, 'Not Taking the Medicine: Sportsmen and Doctors in Late Nineteenth-Century Britain' *Journal of Sport History* 34 (2007), 401–13.

7 R Harland, 'Sport and Exercise Medicine – a personal perspective' *Lancet* 366 (2005), s53–4.

8 House of Commons Committee of Public Accounts, Preparations for the London 2012 Olympic and Paralympic Games (Fiftieth Report of Session 2007–8) (London: HMSO, 2008).

9 The phrase 'ergogenic aid' is broadly defined as anything which enhances physical (and sometimes mental) performance, and as such includes training, hypnosis, drug taking, dietary practices, and so on. R Beamish and I Ritchie, 'From Fixed Capacities to Performance-Enhancing Substances' *Sport in History* 25 (2005), 412–33.

10 These can only be nodded to in footnotes, but as good starting points, see: Beamish and Ritchie, 'From fixed capacities'; P Dimeo, *A History of Drug Use in Sport 1876–1976* (London: Routledge, 2007); Hoberman, *Mortal Engines*; I Van Hilvoorde, R Vos, G de Wert, 'Flopping, Klapping and Gene Doping: Dichotomies Between "Natural" and "Artificial" in Elite Sport' *Social Studies of Science* 37 (2007), 173–200. For a more general history of sports medicine with a very strong emphasis on doping, see I Waddington, 'The Development of Sports Medicine' *Sociology of Sport Journal* 13 (1996), 176–96, and his subsequent work, for example I Waddington and A Smith, *An Introduction to Drugs in Sport, Addicted to winning?* (London: Routledge, 2nd edn, 2008).

11 Hoberman, *Mortal Engines*, p. 9.

12 B Houlihan, Dying to Win: Doping in Sport and the Development of Anti-doping Policy (Strasbourg: Council of Europe, 1999).

13 A Miah, 'From anti-doping to a "performance policy" sport technology, being human, and doing ethics' *European Journal of Sport Science* 5 (2005), 51–7;

B Kayser, A Mauron, A Miah, 'Viewpoint: Legalisation of Performance-enhancing Drugs' *Lancet* 366 (2005), s21; R Beamish and I Ritchie, 'From Chivalrous "Brothers-in-Arms" to the Eligible Athlete: Changed Principles and the IOC's Banned Substance List' *International Review for the Sociology of Sport* 39 (2004), 355–71.

14  Dimeo, A History of Drug Use.

15  For example, the possible risk to health through side-effects, the unsavoury nature of this sexualised invigoration, the crossing of human/animal boundaries, the possibility of coercion, etc. For an earlier period see D Hamilton, *The Monkey Gland Affair* (London: Chatto & Windus, 1986). I would like to thank Dr Hamilton for some information he provided by email in April 2007 about the likely availability of gland extracts in the 1930s.

16  J Goodbody, 'Ready, Steady, Grow: Athletes turn to Viagra', *The Sunday Times*, 22 June 2008; World Anti Doping Agency, *Q&A: 2009 Prohibited List*, www.wada-ama.org/rtecontent/document/QA_List_OR.pdf (accessed August 2009).

17  'Perhaps the greatest untold story in this history is that it was British scientists who established testing procedures for both amphetamines and steroids.' Dimeo, *A History of Drug Use* , p. 14.

18  See the witness statements in LA Reynolds and EM Tansey, The Development of Sports Medicine in Twentieth-Century Britain (Transcript of a Witness Seminar) (London: Wellcome Trust, 2009).

19  J Welshman, 'Only Connect: The History of Sport, Medicine and Society' *International Journal of the History of Sport* 15 (1998), 1–21. Otherwise, see: N Carter, 'Mixing Business with Leisure? The Football Club Doctor, Sports Medicine and the Voluntary Tradition,' *Sport in History* 29 (2009), 69–91; Carter, 'Metatarsals and Magic Sponges: English Football and the Development of Sports Medicine,' *Journal of Sport History* 31 (2007), 53–73; KG Sheard, "Brutal and Degrading': The Medical Profession and Boxing, 1838–1984' *International Journal of the History of Sport* 15 (1998), 74–102; Waddington, 'The Development'; J Berryman & R Park (eds), *Sport and Exercise Science: Essays in the History of Sports Medicine* (Chicago: University of Illinois Press, 1992). There is also a good ethnological and anthropological study of recent sports medicine: P David Howe, *Sport, Professionalism and Pain: Ethnographies of Injury and risk* (London: Routledge, 2004). Otherwise there are some histories of the (non-British) organisations and institutions of sports medicine and science, e.g. S Bailey, *Science in the Service of Physical Education and Sport: The story of the ICSSPE 1956–1996* (Chichester: John Wiley & Sons, 1996); JD Massengale and RA Swanson (eds), *The History of Exercise and Sport Science* (Champaign, Il: Human Kinetics, 1997).

20  For a good example, see 'Chapter 6: The Other Side of Sports Medicine' in Waddington & Smith, *An Introduction to Drugs in Sport*, 83–102, particularly the section 'Sports Medicine: A Brief history', pp. 84–9.

21  See in particular the work of Patricia Vertinsky: P Vertinsky, 'Commentary: What is Sports Medicine?' *Journal of Sport History* 34 (2007), 402–5; Vertinsky,

'Making and Marking Gender: The Medicalization of the Body from One Century's End to Another,' *Culture, Sport and Society* 2 (1999), 1–24; Vertinksy, 'The Social Construction of the Gendered Body: Exercise and the Exercise of Power,' *International Journal of the History of Sport* 11 (1994), 147–71; Vertinsky, 'Old Age, Gender and Physical Activity: The Biomedicalization of Aging,' *Journal of Sport History* 18 (1991), 64–80; Vertinsky, *The Eternally Wounded Woman: Doctors, Women and Exercise in the Late Nineteenth Century* (Manchester: Manchester University Press, 1990) and for her explanation of methodology in this field see Vertinsky, 'Body History for Sport Historians: The Case of Gender and Race' in K Walmesley (ed.), *Method and Methodology in Sport and Cultural History* (Iowa: Brown & Benchmark Publications, 1995), pp. 50–62.

22  Berryman and Park, *Sport and Exercise Science*.

23  There is a bibliography of Park's work in JA Mangan & P Vertinsky, *Gender, Sport, Science: Selected Writings of Roberta J Park* (London: Routledge, 2008).

24  See in particular: RJ Park, '"Mended or Ended?": Football Injuries and the British and American Medical Press, 1870–1910' *The International Journal of the History of Sport* 18 (2001), 110–33; Park, 'High-Protein Diets, 'Damaged Hearts', and Rowing Men: Antecedents of Modern Sports Medicine and Exercise Science, 1867–1928' *Exercise and Sports Science Reviews* 25 (1997), 137–69; Park, 'Athletes and Their Training in Britain and America, 1800–1914' in Berryman and Park, *Sport and Exercise Science*, pp. 57–107; JC Whorton, '"Athlete's Heart": The Medical Debate over Athleticism, 1870–1920' *Journal of Sport History* 9 (1982), 30–52.

25  V Heggie, 'A Century of Cardiomythology: Exercise and the Heart c1880–1980', *Social History of Medicine* 23 (2010), 280–98.

26  Cronin, 'Not taking the medicine'.

27  This project would undoubtedly have looked very different if it had not been for the input of sports historians, particularly Dr Neil Carter, and those attendees at the conferences of the British Society of Sports History who have asked questions and made comments on my work.

28  Good places to start would be: the 'Special Edition: Amateurism in Britain: For the Love of the Game?', *Sport in History* 26 (2006); A Smith and D Porter (eds), *Amateurs and Professionals in Post-war British Sport* (London: Frank Cass, 2000); R Holt & T Mason, *Sport in Britain, 1945–2000* (Oxford: Blackwell, 2000).

29  V Heggie, '"Only the British Appear to be Making a Fuss'; the Science of Success and the Myth of Amateurism at the Mexico Olympiad, 1968' *Sport In History* 28 (2008), 213–35.

30  See Chapter 6 for further discussion of this idea.

31  Sheard, 'Brutal and Degrading'.

32  Anon, 'Gleanings: Footballers and National Insurance' *Athletic News*, 17 June 1912.

33  N Carter, 'Mixing Business with Leisure?' & 'Metatarsals and magic sponges'.

34  Although Physical Culture has tended to be associated more with the fascist

regimes of the early twentieth century, there is work on the British 'super-man' too: I Zweiniger-Bargielowska, 'Building a British Superman: Physical Culture in Interwar Britain' *Journal of Contemporary History* 41 (2006), 595–610. Connecting public health and body image, see D Lupton, *The Imperative of Health: Public Health and the Regulated Body* (London: Sage, 1995), especially Chapter 5 'Bodies, Pleasures and the Practices of the Self', pp. 131–57.

35  F Skillen, '"A sound system of physical training": the development of girls' physical education in interwar Scotland' *History of Education* 38 (2009), 403–18; J Welshman, 'Physical culture and sport in schools in England and Wales, 1900–40' *International Journal of the History of Sport* 15 (1998), 54–75; Welshman, 'Physical Education and the School Medical Service in England and Wales, 1907–1939' *Social History of Medicine* 9 (1996), 31–48; S Fletcher, *Women First: The Female Tradition in English Physical Education, 1880–1980* (London: Athlone Press, 1984).

36  Virginia Berridge identifies 1962 as a crucial year, when the Royal College of Physicians published its report on lung cancer and smoking. V Berridge, 'Medicine, Public Health and the Media in Britain from the Nineteen-fifties to the Nineteen-seventies' *Historical Research* 82 (2009), 360–73; Berridge, 'Medicine and the Public: The 1962 Report of the Royal College of Physicians and the New Public Health' *Bulletin of the History of Medicine* 81 (2007), 286–311.

37  Reynolds and Tansey, The Development of Sports Medicine.

38  Attempts to change the name of BAS(E)M to 'British Association of Sports Sciences and Medicine' in the 1970s, and to 'British Association of Sport, Sciences and Medicine' in the 1980s were unsuccessful. Archives of the British Association of Sport and Exercise Medicine. *Minutes of the Executive Committee*. 29 Mar. 1977; *Secretary's Report*. 22 May 1984.

39  P Bailey, *Leisure and Class in Victorian England: Rational Recreation and the Contest for Control, 1830–1885* (Toronto: University of Toronto Press, 1978); W Baker, 'The leisure revolution in Victorian England: a review of recent literature' *Journal of Sport History* 6 (1979), 76–87; H Cunningham, *Leisure in the Industrial Revolution* (London: Croom Helm, 1980); DE Hall (ed.), *Muscular Christianity: Embodying the Victorian Age* (Cambridge: Cambridge University Press, 1998); B Haley, *The Healthy Body and Victorian Culture* (Harvard: Harvard University Press, 1977); JA Mangan, *Athleticism in the Victorian and Edwardian Public School* (Cambridge: Cambridge University Press, 1981).

40  There is some evidence that women's sport sought out medical and scientific support before men's sport. P Atkinson, 'Strong Minds and Weak Bodies: Sports, Gymnastics, and the Medicalization of women's Education' *British Journal of Sports History* 2 (1985), 62–71; S Fletcher, 'The Making and Breaking of a Female Tradition: Women's Physical Education in England 1880–1980' *International Journal of the History of Sport* 2 (1985), 29–39; J Hargreaves, *Sporting Females: Critical Issues in the History and Sociology of Women's Sports* (London: Routledge, 1994) – see in particular Chapter 4; JA Mangan and RJ Park (eds) *From 'Fair Sex' to Feminism: Sport and the Socialization of Women in*

*the Industrial and Post-Industrial Eras* (London: Routledge, 1987); KE McCrone, 'Play up! Play UP! And Play the Game! Sport at the Late Victorian Girls' Public School' *Journal of British Studies* 23 (1984), 106–34.

41  See Vertinsky cited in footnote 21, above.

42  Not least the development of ergogenic aids, such as amphetamines. See: Dimeo, *A History of Drug Use in Sport*, particularly 'Chapter 4. Amphetamines & Post-war Sport, 1945–1976', pp. 53–68

43  A question which has also been asked by philosophers of sport: F De Wachter, 'The Symbolism of the Healthy Body: A Philosophical Analysis of the Sportive Imagery of Health' *Journal of the Philosophy of Sport* xi (1985), 56–62.

# 2

# Moderate individuals: beginnings, 1900–27

A very good old-fashioned recipe known as 'Black Jack' will not easily be bettered. It takes the form of 1/4lb. Epsom salts, 2 oz. each of bar liquorice, gentian root, camomile flowers, and a little powdered ginger. Place in 2 quarts of water and boil down to 1 quart. Strain through muslin or a fine sieve, and bottle off, adding a little alcoholic spirit (preferably rum or gin) for preservation purposes. Take a large wine-glassful on an empty stomach at night or in the early morning.[1]

In the early decades of the twentieth century, there were no professional sports medicine organisations – no medical organisations dedicated to the needs of sport, and no sporting organisations with dedicated medical sub-committees. Few medical men (and even fewer, if any, medical women) would self-identify as a 'sports doctor' or 'sports surgeon', and the population of specialists in the treatment of sportsmen and women was extremely small. Athletes appeared only rarely as the topics of (or guinea pigs in) papers in biomedical journals. Many sporting events took place without any medical intervention or supervision. With practice and provision so fragmented it is reasonable enough to ask if sports medicine can be said to exist in the early years of the twentieth century. And yet, the recipe quoted above is for a 'detoxing' medicine to be used at the beginning of a training regime, published in 1913, in an athletics training manual available to anyone with interest, literacy and a shilling or two to spare. What can we call this if it is not a form of sports medicine?

When we ask the defining question laid out in the last chapter – 'did the sports participant or athlete get *different* treatment?' – the answer is yes. Much of this is at a very basic level, where injury occurs on the track or field and the athlete gets specially tailored medical first-aid in the first instance. But medical professionals, as well as a large body of laymen, prescribed and proscribed physical activity, injury treatments, pharmaceuticals, dietaries and training regimes. Major sporting events attracted a hard core of voluntary medical attendees, as well as curious physiologists interested in the athletic body; some of these had special medical rules, such as compulsory medical screening or the banning of various drugs. There was even, by the turn of the century, a specialist sports hospital – Matlock House, a.k.a. the 'Footballers' hospital' – in Manchester (see Box 1).

But if we are to make a claim for the existence of sports medicine, it is not enough just to show an abundance of disaggregated practice – it is also necessary to show that these practices shared something in common, that they were part of a wider community of theory and practice. Even without central, controlling bodies or organisations, without specialist journals or training courses, actors in both the medical and sporting spheres were still able to identify some practices as novel or innovative, others as old-fashioned or traditional, and yet more as scientific or mere quackery. What this chapter will go on to show is that both philosophical and physiological theories constrained and informed the construction of sports medicine; these ideas were part of the shared values and liberal education of a generation of middle-class men who, as doctors or amateur athletes, contributed to an understanding of the athletic body in the early twentieth century.

Most importantly this community contained doctors and scientists as well as athletes and coaches. Debates, disagreements and outright controversies were as likely to happen within as between the medical community and the sporting community. Early twentieth-century authors sometimes made a great deal of alleged differences between the strawmen images of superstitious, ignorant coaches pitted against abstracted, elite scientists. Yet such depictions conceal continuity between medicine and sport. Historians have, perhaps, been to ready to take clichés at face value; on closer examination critiques of the old-fashioned coach can be found in the sporting press, while the medical press could round just as quickly on the doctor who was so timid as to suggest that this or that sport might be dangerous.[2]

The athletic body and its medical treatment was circumscribed by understandings of what made a healthy lifestyle, and these were often shared by those trained in medicine as well as the lay population. As shorthand for these ideas I am going to use the words 'moderation' and 'individualism'. Moderation in all things, including diet and exercise, is regularly recommended in training manuals by coaches and doctors alike; meanwhile an individualised approach to exercise was generally promoted, where every would-be athlete needed to attend to the unique demands of his own body. Taken together these ideas can describe appropriate behaviour and activity not just for the body, but also for the mind. This linked healthy physical normality to the character-building aspects of exercise which the leading advocates of Victorian sport had promoted as integral to gentlemanly amateurism.[3]

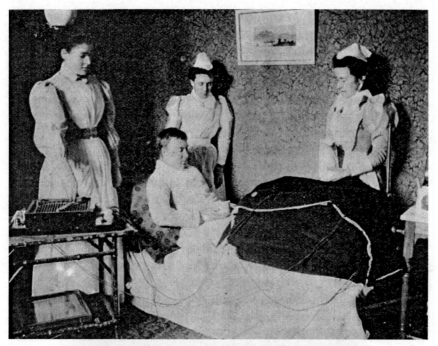

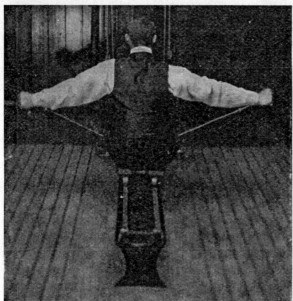

**2.** Various treatments being delivered at the 'Footballers' Hospital', Matlock House in Manchester *c.* 1899. Images taken from M Randal Roberts, 'A Footballers' Hospital', *The Windsor Magazine* (March 1989), 511–16.

These ideas were fully endorsed by contemporary physiological under-standings of the human body, both a traditional Victorian notion of fixity and a newer, emerging, Edwardian understanding of the body as an adapt-able system. In the older physiological paradigm the body is a machine with absolute limits, a fixed store of energy to power both body and mind. Therefore the twin priorities for sport were firstly to avoid overextending the athlete's body, while, secondly, maximising *efficiency* – ensuring that the energy store was used to its best effect. This is the body informed by thermodynamics, where an interest in efficiency and movement in an industrial, productionist, context, bled into research on exercise and sport. Within a generation the pioneering chronophotography of Eadweard Muybridge and Étienne-Jules Marey (both, coincidentally: 1830–1904) was being reproduced in training manuals for athletes.[4] Here movement is broken down into discrete stages which can be individually studied and refigured (as in time and motion studies) allowing the athlete to perfect each part of a sporting action, enabling him to complete a throw or take a stride in the most efficient manner.

Such 'scientific' training was embedded even in the most rigorously 'amateur' of British sports. To take just one example, in the Amateur Rowing Association (ARA; which maintained a fairly high bar for the definition of amateurism, excluding all those who worked on boats and rivers) the discussion of the physics of rowing – angles of blades, forces of elbows, and the design of sliding seats – was a legitimate topic of con-versation. In the 1906–8 logbooks of one Manchester-based ARA club (Agecroft) a satirical essay on coaching, emphasising the 'amateur' nature of the club, is counter-posed a few pages later by an extremely physics-heavy article on 'The Theory and Practice of Belgian Rowing' clipped out of *Yachting and Boating Monthly*.[5]

In the newer, emerging understanding of the human frame, all the bodily systems were vital systems capable of improvement or enhance-ment. Lungs could be expanded, the heart strengthened, the 'wind' increased, flexibility improved, etc. At the beginning of the twentieth century this seems still, at least for sport, to focus on bodies that are sub-par, below normal, or currently unfit. Training manuals took the seden-tary urban worker from winter sloth to competition-ready summer fitness, with the understanding clear that it is the summer state which is normal and natural, while winter sloth is an unnatural feature of civilisation. That the athlete is healthy and normal is emphasised by attitudes towards the use of ergogenic aids, discussed more below. If an athlete felt fatigued he could legitimately reach for the same pharmaceutical products as any other member of society (and they would work just as well for him as for anyone else).

So enhancement could still take place within the confines of the body's normal abilities and limits; it is not until well into the twentieth century that sports doctors seriously begin to talk about manufacturing and creating supernormal performances and enhanced physiques. The obvious exception to this would seem to be the body-builder and strongman, particularly of the Charles Atlas and Eugen Sandow type.[6] It is worth pointing out that these sorts of bodies are not usually depicted as normal, and often not regarded as healthy or 'athletic', by a lay and medical audience alike; their very 'artificial' construction through repetitive movements and exercise are precisely the opposite of the balanced, healthy, vigorous gentleman whose body is the ideal type for this period.[7] To continue with a story partly told; after the satire on coaching and the physics of the Belgian rowing team, Agecroft Rowing Club's log-book has a cutting from the *Manchester Guardian* which mocks the 'unhealthy' body-building craze.[8]

One of the best illustrations of the shift from a fixed to an adaptable understanding of the body is in cardiology where the 'Athlete's Heart' is at first a pathological symptom caused by overextending and straining the heart, and later becomes a healthy physiological (specialist) adaptation which allows the body to safely take part in sport.[9] The Athlete's Heart is one of the few sports-medicine related topics to maintain an almost continual presence in the twentieth-century medical press, as well as courting attention in sporting newspapers and training manuals, as it moves between pathology and physiology. The essence of the problem posed by the Athlete's Heart is the central theme of sports medicine, defining 'normality'. When the athlete was normal, and when enlarged hearts were acknowledged as a symptom of heart disease, then when the athlete presented with an enlarged heart the obvious diagnosis was heart strain (probably caused by exertion). By 1900 a more robust interpretation of the athletic body, as the epitome of the healthy body, determined that normal physical exercise could do no harm to normal bodies; athletes did not have disproportionately enlarged hearts. Therefore, any patients who did have an enlarged heart caused by exercise clearly had a predisposition to heart disease, or a hidden constitutional weakness, or had violated the principle of moderation. Later in the century abnormally large hearts were to become a distinctive, 'normal', physiological feature of the athlete.

### Early sports medicine and its consumers

In a period without obvious organisational or institutional guidelines some key questions are important to the creation of a coherent account of the relationship between sport and medicine. What was sports medicine in this period? Who practised it and where? What did they do, and to what purpose? What theories – biomedical and sporting – was this practice based upon? What was the body upon which sports medicine acted – who or what was the sportsman? What, if anything, made sports medicine different to any other medical or health practices?

As the last chapter argued, there are three types or forms of sports medicine, each with specific aims. Firstly, treatment, much of which is essentially first aid, with the addition of some systems of recovery and rehabilitation. Secondly, there is enhancement; the use of biomedical and biochemical knowledge to alter and improve performance. Finally, there is preventive medicine, often a form of policing which includes attempts to prevent accidents or illness by controlling equipment, playing technique, eligibility to play, etc., as well as the more obvious forms of boundary control such as dope and gender testing. Between the years 1900 and 1927 basic treatment certainly occurred, at all levels from first-aid to specialist interventions (e.g. those at the Footballers' Hospital); enhancement and policing are harder to locate.

Historians have previously argued that the activity that I characterise as enhancement was absent in the early decades of the twentieth century.[10] They argue that athletes and physicians shared an 'ontology of performance' in which the fixed body could not be improved beyond its 'natural limits'. I largely agree, and while I suggest that training manuals and the like did seek to 'improve' the reader, they did so by returning him to healthy normality, and do not seem to seek extra-normal performances. But we should not extrapolate from this to suggest that biomedicine and science was never mobilised to improve performance; they certainly were used, although this may have been used to *reach* limits rather than to *expand* them. So while it is possible – likely even – that many involved in sports continued to use training schemes based on tradition and experience, it is clear from the training manuals, magazines and newspapers of the early twentieth century that some in the world of sport were seeking a scientific 'edge'.

Enhancement brings us to a particular complaint in the history of medicine, which is the invisibility to the historian of many healing practices. Much sports medicine is self-treatment, and often goes unremarked or unrecorded. We may occasionally stumble upon reports of a cyclist's decision to suck barley sugar on a long ride, or a Saturday footballer's use of a home-made poultice for a sprain, but these are exceptions. Likewise, in the area of treatment, practice is usually indistinguishable from other sorts of medical activity, visible and invisible. In this time period, the man arriving at hospital with a fracture of the lower limb caused by a rugby scrum is usually given the same treatment as the one whose leg was broken by a hansom cab. Therefore the one unique site of practice for sports medicine between 1900 and 1927 is usually the one most readily associated with it, and that is the track or field. The answer to the question 'where, uniquely, was sports medicine being practised?' is the athletics track, sports meetings, and the rare (but increasing) number of specialty medical sites such as the operating theatres of knee surgeons or the Footballers' Hospital.

What is perhaps the most distinctive feature of sports medicine at this time is its policing activity; how doctors were able to declare some bodies unfit for some sports – in addition to the 'common sense' decision that women should be excluded from vigorous exercise. In the first decade of the twentieth century this was expressed at the highest competitive levels through the introduction of screening at the Olympic Games. In the same years it was also applied to the lowest level of competitive sport, with extensive discussions over the appropriate duration and format for school sports. Both these issues will be discussed further below.

Who, then, was practising these three areas of sports medicine? Any such practitioners were by-and-large voluntary or privately supplied; outside of school sports there was no state involvement to speak of (which is entirely consistent with the state of medicine in Britain at the turn of the century). Sports medicine practitioners were often involved by accident (in both senses of the word), such as the Liverpool surgeon who came down from the stands to treat his injured son at a rugby match in 1907.[11] Some sports medics were more regular volunteers, like members of the St John Ambulance, who attended many of the largest athletic and sporting meets. There were also enthusiasts, often (ex)sportsmen themselves who actively sought out opportunities to work with athletes. (A classic example is Adolphe Abrahams, discussed in Box 2). Finally there were the rare, but growing, band of specialists who made a living from dealing with sportsmen and sports clubs – for example J Ward, a surgeon, whose advert in the *Athletic News* in 1907 claimed that he was

> England's greatest bloodless surgeon ... The man with a gift that is outclassing medical skill in Manchester and Bolton [who] can save Insurance Companies and the Football Clubs thousands of pounds, as he has the greatest percentage of absolute cures in England.[12]

Sports medicine was not limited to doctors and surgeons; workers in the professions allied to medicine, particularly masseurs, contributed to the practice of sports medicine, alongside truly amateur medics such as autodidact coaches and trainers.

What is particularly evident is that sports medicine between 1900 and

1927 is in places a highly commercialised activity. The commercialisation of sport is more usually located in the middle of the twentieth century (coinciding with being televised), but by 1900 sports medicine was part of a vibrant medical market place.[13] In training manuals patent medicine jostled for advertising space with dietary supplements and specialist healers. The cachet of sport – healthy and manly – was a useful tool for advertisers. A quick survey of adverts in the *Athletic News* around 1900 shows sports being used to sell Vi-Cola and Cadbury's cocoa, while the New Zealand rugby team endorse the use of Zam-Buk muscle embrocation. Likewise, Albert Trott 'The Popular Middlesex Cricketer, Explains to the British Public the remarkable Curative Effect of Electricity, the Modern Wonder-Worker'.[14] Training manuals, coaching pamphlets, and the services of the bloodless surgeon J Ward were all advertised using testimonials from more and less famous sportsmen.

Such associations between commercial interests and sports did not stop with straightforward advertising; the apparently profitable business of sponsoring sporting events also took place in the early twentieth century. At the first London Olympiad in 1908 the marathon was effectively sponsored by Oxo, who were appointed by the British Olympic Association as the 'official caterers'.[15] Oxo representatives were available at several points along the marathon, supplying (free of charge to runners) an 'Oxo Athletes' Flask, containing Oxo for immediate use', as well as 'Oxo hot and cold; Oxo and Soda, Rice Pudding, raisins, Bananas, Soda and Milk'.[16] Oxo was, of course, a scientific dietary product, promoted as much for its nutritional and health benefits as for taste, convenience and cost. Furthermore, the Oxo representatives had an explicitly medical role, since, as well as Oxo, they also provided '[s]timulants ... in case of collapse' and 'Eau de Cologne and sponges' for the same purpose.[17]

Much of this commercialised medicine, a tub of Zam-buk or a mug of Oxo, was within the means of many would-be athletes. Other products and services were less accessible, such as the specialist surgical treatment, or the advice to take up an expensive high-protein diet, or to rest completely from work to repair a sprain. This is not to say that all sports medicine was consumer medicine, or that all of it was paid for by the patient. As mentioned above, St John Ambulance staff were sometimes available at sporting events for the immediate provision of first aid, and transport to a local hospital or doctor. Yet their presence was not guaranteed, as reports of mid-sized sporting events show:

[A] nasty accident occurred in the quarter-mile obstacle race. Ralph Clayton of Bollington Harriers, dropping awkwardly over a hurdle and spraining an ankle. As there were no ambulance men on the ground, it was some little time before assistance could be obtained, Clayton, in the meantime, suffering much pain.[18]

Free treatment, especially in the form of first aid, was also available from the 'enthusiasts' – doctors (and in the case of university teams, student doctors) who offered their time to, or were members of, sports clubs.

Some sports medicine was bought for the sportsman. Although the club doctor, waiting in the dressing room or in the stands at large football matches, may have been an unpaid volunteer, the army of medical specialists who treated footballers were not. Even a cursory perusal of the sporting press of the period will uncover a list of 'crocked' athletes/sportsmen, all of whom appear to be getting specialist treatment.[19] In the richest and most popular professional sport, Association Football, players in the wealthier teams could clearly expect attendance by multiple practitioners and affiliated medical services, such as massage, and, where necessary, extensive hospitalisations, rehabilitation, time in private clinics and the attention of Harley Street specialists.

Where a club could not run to such costly treatment, or in the case of amateur players not covered by insurance, medical services could still be provided by public donation or the actions of individual benefactors. Such treatment was not limited to medical intervention for strictly sports-related conditions:

> Old Lancashire players and the present day supporters of the team will regret to learn that Frank Ward has been remitted to an inebriates' home near Gloucester for the next twelve months ... Mr. John Allison ... has taken a deep interest in the case ... and made himself responsible for the £40 required for his maintenance in the home – before he knew whether any help would be forthcoming. On Friday, the Lancashire County Cricket Club voted a donation of £10, Mr H.J. Maden has subscribed £5, and 'Anonymous' has forwarded £1 to the Editor of this paper.[20]

## The Olympics and international sports medicine

The patchy medical services at local and national events were outclassed by the provision at international level, although medical services at such events present significant logistical challenges to organisers. The regulated and team-based Olympic Games of the twentieth century took several Olympiads to emerge; though British competitors were present in 1896 at Athens, in 1900 at Paris, in St Louis in 1904 and at the unofficial 'intercalated' games in Athens once more in 1906, they were present more as a self-motivated set of individuals rather than a coherent team.

Furthermore, there were extremely limited funds available to athletes to cover their travel. Food and accommodation was usually free or subsidised for competitors, but there continued to be some difficulty with the nature and definition of amateurism within the Olympics, with confusion existing over whether this sort of subsidy could technically count as payment for competing (thus rendering all attendees automatically professionals, disqualifying them before they could even get on the track). In 1906, potential competitors in the cycling events were asked by the National Cycling Union representative to pay £15 up-front to cover accommodation, travel, food, etc.[21] So the majority of those who attended the early Olympics did so under their own steam. This clearly excluded all but the moderately wealthy, meaning many of those who attended could well afford their own medical treatment too.

We can first consider the British competitors at the Olympic Games as a coherent team in 1908. The British Olympic Association (BOA) was formed in 1905, in time to co-ordinate and plan the London Games of 1908. Medical provision followed the pattern of previous and subsequent Olympics, relying heavily on voluntary services from St John Ambulance and individual medical professionals, supplemented by military assistance. There was no Olympic village in 1908 – this system was first pioneered in 1932 at the Los Angeles Games – and so the more than two thousand competitors (2,022, with just 44 women) were housed in guest houses and hotels, which were either recommended by the BOA, or sourced by the visiting teams themselves, the American team choosing to stay in Brighton, for example.[22] Therefore there was no central location for medical provision other than at the stadium itself, and most teams either brought their own attendees or bought the services of doctors and hospitals if necessary.

The 1908 marathon certainly had some medical supervision, above and beyond the Oxo representatives. The official report of the Games lists seven 'Medical Attendants and Examiners' for the marathon, six of whom have the title 'Dr'. Regulations concerning the marathon also indicate that medical professionals, appointed by the BOA, were going to patrol the course; such activity had been undertaken since the first modern games in 1896, where the marathon runners were followed by doctors in carts.[23] The marathon was a relatively dramatic event, with the Italian runner Pietri overtaking the American Hefferson in the last mile, but collapsing on entering the stadium. Pietri collapsed several times, and was looked after by 'doctors and attendants' who ended up effectively carrying him over the finish line.[24] A great controversy ensued between the BOA and the American delegation, and Pietri's gold medal was eventually revoked and first place was awarded to Hefferson.

Another controversy hints at medical supervision for team games; accused of illegally wearing spikes the Australian Rugby Captain – himself a doctor – claimed in his autobiography that he 'insisted at once on an examination of the boots of all the players as they came off the field at full time, and [he] nominated an English doctor to carry out the task'.[25] On the other hand, it can also be inferred that medical supervision was certainly not blanket; in the heats for the high diving a British competitor became unconscious after a dive and had to be rescued and assisted by a co-competitor from Sweden.[26] Whatever the medical provision supplied by the organisers, only one sport had its medical staff formally listed in the official report, and that was Gymnastics, whose (honorary) medical attendees included a JA Howard Esq. MD, and Surgeon Bell, RN.[27] This lack of formal records is deceptive; the British Olympic team did have a medical attendant in 1908 and 1912, as Adolphe Abrahams attended with the track and field team (his brother Harold Abrahams was a team member). Medical attendance increased, with several sports taking their own masseurs, etc., although it was not until 1928 (Amsterdam) that the BOA officially appointed a medical officer to attend to the whole team.

Of all the sporting events it was the marathon that received more than its share of medical attention. The marathon was also the first event whose conduct and timing was altered according to the advice of medical experts. There are two reasons for this concentration; first, the pragmatic and reactive – the marathon was the first Olympic event in which a competitor died. This was despite the fact that at this particular Olympics, in Stockholm, 1912, relatively extensive (when we compare supply to demand) medical provision was made for both athletes and spectators.[28] Medical supervision for events outside the stadium were arranged by the relevant sports governing bodies, namely athletics, swimming, rowing, cycling, fencing and horse-riding.Within the stadium three rooms were provided, with beds and operating equipment, permanently staffed by at least two doctors, five attendants and two nurses. Similarly, the provision for the marathon was extensive; five medical stations, all bar one with a bed, staffed by a doctor and three to six further staff, with an ambulance and a range of equipment including stimulants and stretchers. One medical station also offered drinking water, and the course was attended by nine patrols of Boy Scouts also equipped with water and signalling flags. The total attendance at the marathon included twenty medical professionals (doctors, nurses and attendants), and thirty other volunteers. But, as the official report states 'in spite of all this the marathon race . . . was to cost a human life'.[29]

The Portuguese runner, Francesco Lazaro collapsed during the race, and was attended on the track by two doctors; he was removed to hospital and treated for sunstroke, but died the following morning.[30] Three other competitors in the marathon were also diagnosed with sunstroke. After the event, the seven doctors in attendance on rotation at the Stadium wrote a letter-cum-report to the IOC, recommending that if the marathon were to continue to be part of the Olympic programme, it ought to be scheduled only for the coolest part of the day.[31] The IOC had at this time no medical committee or such like to make (or ratify) such recommendations, but the suggestions of the Stockholm doctors were adhered to for all future Olympic marathons.

The cancellation of subsequent Olympiads because of World War I meant that it was several years before this medical advice was heeded, but when the Olympics restarted in 1920 the medical support to the marathon was increased, and the event was scheduled for the afternoon. This was a pragmatic and reactive response to medical advice, but there was also a *preventive*, proactive medical response to the biological stresses and strains of the marathon. By 1908 and 1912 athletes who wanted to take part in the marathon and the cycling events, respectively, had to be medically screened to ensure that they were healthy enough to take part in elite sport. These events were singled out because they were apparently those which posed the greatest challenge to the body, according to contemporary understandings of human physiology. So although team sports (particularly Rugby and Association Football) and boxing cropped up as objects of criticism in the medical press, it was the endurance sports which elicited practical medical intervention.

## Moderation in all things

The changes in theories and laws describing the workings of the 'human motor' in the nineteenth century are discussed elsewhere, and need not be repeated here.[32] By the turn of the twentieth century there were at least two widely used metaphors available to describe the human body at work and at play. In one construction – the most longstanding – the body was a fixed and stable machine, whose inputs and outputs were in careful balance, which had a specific capacity for work, and largely unalterable limits. In the other, newer, understanding, the human body was an adaptable and vital machine capable of enhancement and change to fit its environment. Alongside these contemporary understandings of the body I have suggested that notions of moderation and individualism could be used by athletes and doctors to assess biomedical claims about treatments and training regimes.

Moderation, meaning an even-handed, sanguine, temperate and

emotionally continent approach to life, is the most obvious interpretation of a well-balanced machine body; moreover, it is a clearly moral imperative, dictating the appropriate attitude towards athletic participation.[33] Over-exertion – pushing the human body beyond its natural limits – therefore posed both a moral and a direct physical danger to the athlete. The moral danger lay in the possibility of becoming 'obsessed' with one's sport, to the neglect of one's other interests, and/or risking psychological harm through over-reacting to losses and wins. The physical danger lay, in its most common aspect, in 'staleness' (see Box 3). In its most extreme form exertion beyond the body's inherent capabilities led to permanent disability and even death.

Training texts repeat the dictum of *moderation* relentlessly. It can be applied to specific aspects of athletic training, or be a generalist rule-of-thumb.[34] The *Athletic News'* own training manual insisted that 'moderation in all things should be the maxim for all men who go into training'.[35] Likewise Adolphe Abrahams argued that '[a] regular system and moderation in all things form the bases of all methods of training and physical culture' going on to emphasise that:

> [n]o two men are alike mentally or bodily, in their habits or peculiarities, and it is therefore impossible and absurd that any definite set of training rules and regulations can possibly be sufficient or suitable for a large number of differently constituted athletes.[36]

As the *Athletic News'* sports medicine expert concisely stated in 1908: '[m]y final word in this connection is, do everything in moderation, and nothing in excess'.[37]

Moderation is both practice and ideology, and it is also supremely flexible; for example, the injection of just one or two doses of strychnine to 'pep up' a long distance runner might be moderate – or we might consider the use of any sort of stimulant as evidence of an immoderate, over-competitive attitude.[38] Moderation had the advantage of a basis in sound, even elite, science and medicine, yet at the same time was extremely pragmatic and easy to apply 'in the field'. Since a definition of moderation was not explicit, it could vary from athlete to athlete, coach to coach, and doctor to doctor; it also provided an easy critique of any competing training regimen – these needed simply to be declared 'immoderate'. Moderation even acted as a protective barrier between the more vigorous or violent contact sports and the criticism of the medical profession. Although at the turn of the century the medical press sometimes carried articles condemning the number of injuries occurring during Rugby or Association Football, their criticisms were never of the game itself – to call for a ban would, of course, be immoderate.[39] Instead what is criticised is the *immoderate* play of the participants (usually inspired by over-competitiveness and financial rewards); Football in the ideal remains a normal, even health-giving and character building, activity.

Moderation's enduring rhetorical value cannot be accounted for merely through its rootedness in contemporary physiology. In the specific world of sport what moderation tied most closely to was the nebulous concept of 'amateurism' which, as previously discussed, has been a powerful trope not only in the *history* of British sports, but also, and possibly more importantly, in *histories* of British sport. There is rarely an appropriate or definitive explanation of amateurism available to the historian, except in extremely specific circumstances – such as where it is defined as a category or requirement of membership for a particular club. Even the IOC, perhaps the ultimate global arbitrator of international amateurism, has rarely defined the term, preferring instead to rely on the various differing guidelines of national governing bodies of sport.

What makes amateurism so slippery is its existence as both practice and ideology. In practice it is most simply the undertaking of sport without financial reward – though, of course, what a 'financial reward' consists of can be variably interpreted. As an ideology, amateurism embodies things which appear to follow on from, or dictate, play without pay; playing for the love of the sport (not fame or money) and scrupulously fair play (the point being to compete, not to win). Amateurism is most commonly interpreted through a class-focused methodology. Simply put, the amateur is a (gentle)man who can literally 'afford' to participate in sport without need of financial recompense. He is also, presumably, of such sensibility that he can avoid overt displays of competitiveness or aggression.

Moderation/amateurism did not function alone; one of the dangers of team games, and one of the reasons why a 'moderate' player might be driven to immoderation, was the loss of that other trope of sporting theory, 'individualism'. Aside from assertions about moderation, what a great many recommended dietaries, training regimes, systems of exercise, massage schedules, etc., all had in common was the inclusion of a cautionary note that '[w]e are not all built one way'.[40] Although human bodies may have been machines, ruled and regulated by physical and mathematical laws, they were not identical. While some of these differences were put down to psychological factors, it was also believed that there were physical differences between athletes. So 'individualism' was both a physical or biomedical practice, and a moral or mental characteristic. It could encourage moderation and protect against the danger of overstrain; it was when an athlete forgot himself and his limits, egged on by a team or a desire to glorify school or country, that he was most in danger of exceeding his natural limitations.

The prioritisation of the uniqueness of the individual was also a mechanism by which certain practices could be condemned as quackery or faddism. By advocating a single scheme as suitable for all, whether it was a high-protein diet, teetotalism, or skipping as exercise, would-be spokesmen could be dismissed as cranks or obsessives, 'addicted' to their own system(s). Indeed, such schemes, because they were immoderate and did not take account of the individual's assumed physical limitations, were not just useless but could actually be dangerous. For example, one cautionary tale in the *Athletic News* read:

> Some little time ago there appeared a number of articles in popular publications recommending rope-skipping as a universal remedy and health preserver. Directions were laid down that skipping for half an hour or an hour at a stretch should be indulged in two or three times a day after meals, just as if it were taken as medicine, but nothing was mentioned with respect to individuals to whom rope-skipping might be injurious ... One young girl suffered from anaemia and heart-weakness died within a short time after rope-skipping for a week in accordance with instructions.[41]

Individualism, like moderation, allowed for an extremely flexible mainstream of exercise science and sporting advice. While the author of a training book might not dare to recommend vegetarianism to all, which would be immoderate and non-individual, he would also avoid condemning it as a system because, presumably, there must be at least one individual for whom it would work.[42] Individualism and moderation therefore also highlight which sports were particularly dangerous, and, significantly, are used both by the medical and the sporting press. The marathon, though a highly individual undertaking, was clearly immoderate. Association Football and Rugby required an individual to think of the team before themselves, and peer pressure might cause immoderate activity. Some sports were doubly dangerous; rowing required not only extreme exertion, but also dictated the absolute loss of individualism to the rhythm of the team.

Individualism and moderation also identified which bodies were particularly vulnerable to the dangers of sport. As a consequence of debates about national fitness, the early twentieth century saw a renewed interest in the types of compulsory physical education to be provided in schools, and hence discussion of school sports and schoolboys. At this time most school-based physical education consisted largely of drill; partly due to lack of resources and space for game playing or running in working class areas. Further, these discussions were explicitly about schoolboys; cross-country running was practically *verboten* for young women and girls.[43]

The inability to comprehend one's individuality, to understand one's limits and act moderately is essentially a moral weakness. As such it was regularly suggested that schoolboys were particularly vulnerable to immoderate sporting behaviour. Cheered on by team-mates, pushing themselves to achieve victory for their school, boys' bodies were thought to be extremely vulnerable to overstress and overstrain. This intimate connection between moral and physical weakness, this belief that moral failings would appear as physical stigmata was a strong and pervasive hangover from Victorian theories of the mind/body continuum.[44]

The link between mental and physical exertion is also reflected in the thermodynamically informed fixed system theories of physiology discussed at the beginning of this chapter. As such, brain and brawn draw upon the same source of energy, which poses a particular challenge to the university student or the schoolchild. Equally, this characterisation could be utilised to explain the 'nervous energy' of an athlete – it was the displacement of physical energy.

> A man's total energy has a limit both in mind and muscle. If nearly all his nervous energy is used up on his motor centres there is little left for the psychical or intellectual part of his brain ... So it often happens that the young athlete becomes eminent for energy and mental activity in after life. The nervous energy has been there and continues there, but is diverted then from muscle to mind.[45]

In 1909 the *British Medical Journal (BMJ)* gave extensive coverage to a debate on the dangers of cross-country running by schoolboys, in which all the aspects of sport as a paradox – a physical and moral danger as well as a source of physical and moral growth – were explicitly discussed. One of the eminent doctors who initiated this debate about school sports, Sir Lauder Brunton (1844–1916), summarised these arguments in his evidence to the Medical Officers of Schools Association:

> Physical exercise of one kind or another is absolutely necessary for boys, in order to ensure their proper development, and that boys must be so occupied as to prevent them becoming loafers. Exercise within bounds tends to increase the power of the muscles, of the lungs, of the heart, and of the nervous system. The discipline of games is of the highest utility in training boys to obedience, self-sacrifice, bravery, alertness, and decision, and teaches them how to acquire command over themselves first and then over others.[46]

Brunton, who was primarily a pharmacologist, in the same evidence also makes specific note of the principles of moderation and of individualism – knowing one's own limits. As he put it 'I am anxious not to prevent [sports] but to regulate them'.[47] Key here, too, was the flexibility of the boy's body; trainable (morally and physically), and adaptable.

The debates over which sports were safe, and for whom, were part of a much larger set of ambiguities in sports medicine. While certain fitness and training practices seem to have remained at the very margins of acceptable activity – such as vegetarianism or teetotalism – others appeared much more mainstream. Massage, high-protein or high-carbohydrate diets, hot or cold baths, rest periods, etc., were used to some degree or another in most sports, both professional and amateur, but their relative importance and exact application seems to have been constantly debated. That some practices were taken up, some maintained, and some dismissed, poses a question about authority in sports medicine. Even without organisations, institutions or certificates there was clearly a mechanism, albeit informal, by which sportsmen and their coaches invested confidence in the judgement of one advocate or another.

Where, then, was authority invested in early twentieth-century sports medicine? The authority of professionals, particularly physicians and scientists, but also successful athletes and coaches, was often invoked. It is misleading to assume that the lack of a professional qualification is evidence for a lack of interest in or engagement with biomedicine; it is clear that some sportsmen took it upon themselves to become amateur medics and physiologists. An article about the Football Hospital in Manchester notes that:

> [t]he Aston Villa captain is great on patent medicines and medical knowledge generally. He has all sorts of cures of his own for every sort of ailment and learnedly discourses with his physician on the merits of all new-fangled cures.[48]

Experience was clearly valued, and the training schemes of the successful sportsman or coach and the treatment of the experienced doctor were in great demand.

But neither professional experience nor athletic success were sufficient in and of themselves. For example, in 1909, '[a]t the instigation of a well-known Footballer . . . half-a-dozen eminent members of [the medical] profession whose *ipse dixit* alone was almost sufficient for . . . unchallenged acceptance' wrote to the *Times* to heavily criticise boys' involvement with cross country running.[49] Their claim was that races over a mile were 'wholly unsuitable for boys under the age of nineteen'.[50] Despite their apparent eminence, an investigation by the Medical Officers of Schools Association and several studies published in the medical press disputed and disproved this suggestion.[51]

Likewise athletic success was no guarantee of authority; Eustace Miles, racquets and tennis champion of the early 1900s, advocated a vegetarian system, published his own cook books, marketed a range of patent food and cooking equipment, and even opened a restaurant. His qualifications as a sportsman did not, however, protect him from counter-claims of faddism or eccentricity in his dietary recommendations.[52] Thus theories of sports medicine in the early twentieth century were informed and swayed by athletic experience and sporting ethics, but remained grounded in contemporary physiological theories of mind and body.

There is a tension between experience and experiment in sports medicine. The adoption and use of any training or treatment scheme can be conceptualised as an experiment; although anything that obviously violated the principles of moderation or individualism would probably be suspect, most diets, exercise routines and therapeutic interventions were ultimately judged by their outcomes as much as their relationship to the 'theory' of training or sports medicine. At the same time individual athletes could not afford to be too experimental, particularly the professionals. With only a short career many were unwilling to give up on tried-and-tested systems in favour of new schemes, however persuasive the theory which backed them up. Indeed, this tendency to stick to the familiar was part-and-parcel of the rhetoric of moderation – sudden changes to lifestyle or environment were warned against, including the sudden return to vigorous exercise after the off season. Change and disruption were a rather repetitive explanation for the poor performance of British teams overseas, especially at the Olympics, where everything from the weather to the food was blamed for the underperformance of competitors.[53]

The would-be sports medicine expert, both the doctor and the athlete, had to create a balance between tradition and modernity. Training regimes could be criticised as quickly for their fashionable uptake of the latest 'fad' as they could for sticking too rigidly to old-fashioned systems and dietary regimes (or 'dietaries'). We also need to recognise the use of the 'old-fashioned' or 'traditional' training regime as another strawman (alongside the cliché of the superstitious coach and cautious doctor); the scientific illiteracy and unpleasantness of the 'traditional' regime is included to reflect a better light upon the authors' preferred 'modern' system. Park has claimed that the 'traditional' high-protein, low-liquid diet (the typical format being steak, stale bread and severe water restriction) of the professional boxer or pedestrian (long-distance walker) of the early nineteenth century was followed 'long after science had confirmed the merits of other regimens'.[54] Yet it is hard to find a training manual published after 1850 which does not cite this practice as old-fashioned, usually dismissing it in favour of what are claimed to be more 'scientific' dietaries. By 1902 the *Athletic News'* own training manual claimed that '[t]he old "rule of thumb" style of dieting – half-cooked meat in large quantities with little else to accompany it but stale bread . . . has long since been exploded'.[55]

Significantly, much of this criticism disguises the fact that these 'rule of thumb' dietaries were themselves based on the science and medicine of the day. One of the major justifications for the stale-bread diet was the avoidance of indigestion and stomach trouble during training and competition, which continues into the twenty-first century as a key feature of most suggested athletic dietary regimes.[56] Park may be right that some, or many, or maybe even most athletes active around 1900 pursued a similar, traditional, sporting diet, but we can expect to find little evidence to prove or disprove her assertion of what was eaten in practice, or how widespread the stale-bread diet really was. What we can say for sure is that the authors of training manuals certainly saw the propaganda value of claiming that they were describing scientific dietaries and that their training regimes coincided completely with contemporary medical thought. There is a strong argument to be made here that some of this rhetoric was a function of a change in the class of athletes, from working-class professionals to a vastly expanded field of middle-class Victorian and Edwardian practitioners. 'Scientific' training was a useful marker of difference between the bodies of the underclass and the bodies of the new, late nineteenth-century athlete. This is a theory too large to be given space here, but is being developed elsewhere.[57]

## Massage, movement and modernity

The prevalence and uptake of 'scientific' training and medical treatment can be best illustrated by two examples, the use of exercise as a cure, and of 'scientific' massage in sport. The use of exercise as a curative therapy is bound up with the histories of massage, physiotherapy, passive movement, medical gymnastics and all allied treatments such as hydrotherapy or electrotherapy. Most of these have roots reaching at least to classical Greek or Roman medicine, and all experienced a boom in popularity towards the end of the nineteenth century. The opposed systems of rest and exercise as treatments for any disease – we concentrate here on orthopaedics; sprains, strains and fractures – are variously supported and dismissed in medical journals and textbooks through the whole of the twentieth century. While the trope of early exercise and movement has generally been favoured, very different definitions of 'early' and 'exercise' exist, and study and counter-study have produced sometimes ambiguous results.[58] What is significant for our story, however, is how frequently the idea of exercise was associated with modernity.

The cases for both rest and exercise were popularly made in the second half of the nineteenth century. For rest the seminal work was by James Hilton, the famous physiologist and surgeon, titled *Rest and Pain* and originally published between 1860 and 1863 as a series of lectures in the *Lancet*.[59] *Rest and Pain* did not concentrate on orthopaedic illness, or sports medicine of any sort, but rather made the case for pain as a diagnostic tool, and rest as a therapy. As such, it fitted neatly with the 'fixed' physiological conception of the body; if energy is needed to repair and heal the body, then it needs to be 'freed up' by reducing energy demands from other body systems. The alternatives, massage and movement, were particularly promoted by the publication of the influential book *Massage and Mobilisation in the Treatment of Fractures* by French surgeon Lucas-Championère in 1889.[60]

With the increasing popularity of medical massage and remedial gymnastics, British doctors began to experiment with, and recommend, massage and exercise (both passive and active movement) in cases of orthopaedic injuries. For example, in 1898 William Bennett, a London surgeon, published an extensive article in the *Lancet* on 'The Use of Massage in the treatment of Recent Fractures', which stated that:

> [t]he usual method of treating facture by prolonged retention of the affected limb in splints which allow of practically no movement of the soft parts about the fracture . . . leads to a large percentage of the unsatisfactory results which follow upon fractures especially in the vicinity of joints.[61]

Two years later, in 1900, Bennett again published an article in the *Lancet* on massage repeating his arguments; '[m]y main object is to urge upon you the desirability of shaking off to some extent the incubus of the traditional routine treatment of fractures . . . prolonged splinting, strappings, counter-irritants, &c'.[62] By 1902 another correspondent to the *Lancet* dismissed 'the Plaster-of-Paris treatment' as 'barbarous'.[63]

By 1909, absolute (i.e. immoderate) rest was already being described as a therapy of the past:

> In the past too much stress has been laid on the importance of rest in cases of injury, and it is largely to the French school that the credit is due of accentuating the importance of the other great factors in treatment, movement and exercise.[64]

Movement and modernity were intimately related. 'The axiom underlying the whole of the [exercise] treatment is that 'movement is life" wrote another doctor in the *Lancet* in 1913.[65] Despite this support a 'fractures committee' of the British Medical Association which reported in 1913, was unable to come to a unanimous conclusion in favour of exercise treatment; this was apparently because mobilisation had been misunderstood and misused so that the practice had been unfairly 'obscured and so discredited'.[66]

The advent of war in the following year led to a new urgency for rapid, functional healing of injuries, especially orthopaedic ones. The increased use of systems of active treatment, including exercise, massage and heat therapy, were transferred into civilian practice at the end of the conflict.[67] In subsequent years articles on 'rest vs. exercise' almost always contained a reference to the 'bad old days' where patients were immobilised for strains, sprains and fractures.[68] In Dr RS Woods' autobiographical account of his experience of sports medicine in the early twentieth century, he blames Hilton for the premature ending of his own sporting career:

> [w]hen I was seventeen [1909], I had hoped to be in the Dulwich XI, as well as the XV, for two seasons. But a sprained ankle one summer and 'water-on-the-knee' the next effectively blighted my cricketing ambitions – thanks to the useless treatment of those days, when Hilton's classic 'Essays on Rest and Pain' . . . had set the clock back for many years to come.[69]

So where did sports medicine stand with regard to rest *versus* exercise? Woods claimed to have introduced mobilisation, 'disregarding the contemporary "masterly inactivity"', in the 1920s, inspired by the publication of a paper by Frank Romer in 1923.[70] Romer was surgeon to the Jockey Club and Honorary Surgeon to the Royal Academy of Music (and was therefore in a position to see a great number of orthopaedic and repetitive strain injuries). Published in *The Practitioner* in 1923, Romer's 'Sports Injuries' is probably the first comprehensive account of sports-related disabilities in the British medical press.[71] This would locate sports medicine's adoption of early exercise after World War I, i.e. *after* its popularisation in mainstream medicine.

However, if we turn to the *sporting* press it appears that early exercise, and movement as therapy, had actually had a much longer history in sports medicine. The *Athletic News* carried a series of articles called 'Medical Miscellany' in the early years of the twentieth century, written by Dr J Ker Lindsay, Honorary Medical Officer to Chelsea Football Club. In *every* column on orthopaedic diseases, from sprains to fractures, Lindsay advocates some sort of active movement in treatment. In the case of the Footballer's knee he states that 'splints [i.e. immobilisation] should never

be used'.[72] With regard to sprained ankles, '[p]rolonged rest is only mentioned to be condemned'.[73] The only exception to this advice is synovitis
of the knee, which was, in his opinion, treated with baths and exercise *too
early* – evidence that early exercise was practised by other medical men in
connection with sports injuries.[74] Later, in 1910, the *Athletic News'* new
medical columnist ('APP') pointed out that while most sprains used to be
treated with 'perfect rest . . . now we go to the other extreme'.[75]

Lest we assume that such practices were limited to just professional
football, similar advice was given in training manuals for amateur athletics. Indeed in some cases footballers may have been subject to more
enforced rest than other athletes, as they were often said to be keen to
get back to work, and unwilling to 'take it easy'. The Footballers' Hospital
dealt with the problem of over-keen footballers (and those who wished to
leave the teetotal institution and visit the local public house) via:

> a machine [fitted] to the patient's leg which . . . keep[s] the knee in constant
> movement . . . [and which] serves the double purpose of helping to heal the
> knee and . . . [curbing] the wearer's propensity to roam.[76]

Albeit not in quite the same format as Woods' treatment of the 1920s and
1930s, this 'wily contrivance' is at least an acknowledgement of the utility
of movement as treatment in sports medicine even before 1900.[77]

Early mobilisation in the treatment of fractures often went hand-in-
hand with the use of massage, especially after the publication of *Massage
and Mobilisation* in 1889. Massage, too, was part of a series of inter-related
treatments, interventions and professions, and the twentieth century saw
the merging and expansion of several of the British societies of massage,
remedial/medical gymnastics and physiotherapy.[78] Although absolutely
ignored in current histories of sports medicine that focus on enhancement and doping, masseurs and physiotherapists were among the first
specialists in sports medicine; by the 1950s professional physiotherapy
organisations were asserting their right to be the sole official providers of
care to sports clubs.

The first professional massage organisation in Britain was formed in
1894 – the Society of Trained Masseuses – as a consequence of three
major influences. Firstly, the increasing medical (and lay) interest in
massage, movement, hydrotherapy, etc.; secondly, the presence of a new
demographic of middle-class women seeking work; thirdly, an increasing
desire, present in many medical disciplines, to form professional societies
to distinguish between 'quacks' and regular practitioners. The last straw
for the profession of massage was the 'Massage Scandal' of 1894, where
an article in the *BMJ* about brothels masquerading as massage houses led
to a special Scotland Yard investigation.[79]

In the early years of the century massage was available in a limited number of hospitals and medical institutions; those individuals with sufficient funds could also buy the services of a masseur/euse – qualified or unqualified, to be taken independently (in the cases of the formally unqualified) or under medical instruction (in the case of those who were members of the Society of Trained Masseuses). It was World War I which raised the profile of massage – the mobilisation of a large army for long-term warfare brought to the fore issues which had previously been of more significance in sports medicine than in general practice, such as the rehabilitation of the injured. Massage and physiotherapy played a prominent role in the schemes of rehabilitation for injured soldiers, returning them to the front during conflict, and to economically productive jobs after 1918.[80]

The athlete's body is superficially like the soldier's body; young, male and 'fit'. However in the medical accounts of the work of masseurs and physiotherapists in the early twentieth century, before World War I, there is little or no reference to massage for athletes. We might well interpret this as evidence for a lack of interest or practice in sports medicine in Britain. Yet, just as sports had quietly been using exercise therapy rather than rest, so it had also been using massage, not only in the treatment and rehabilitation of sportsmen but also in their preparation and training. Massage had also become a rhetoric of modernity in sports, with the 'old fashioned' rubber played off against the well-informed masseur. 'Rubbers' have a long history in British sports, accompanying many of the famous pedestrians of the nineteenth century, as well as boxers and rowers; 'rubber', coach or trainer, team manager, and promoter were often one and the same person. The duty of a 'rubber' – a brisk rub down with a rough towel before and/or after competition – is clearly indicated in the name.[81]

But to engage the newly professionalised masseurs, sporting organisations, sportsmen and sports teams had to overcome two significant hurdles. First and foremost was gender; professional massage was an overwhelmingly female activity as full membership of the Society of Trained Masseuses was open only to women until 1920, and only a very select few men could even qualify to take the examination.[82] Further, the Society of Trained Masseuses had a rule that no 'general' massage should be given by its (female) members upon men – and by 'general' what was meant was exactly the sort of rubbing down and warming up athletes needed; likewise their rule not to act except under 'medical direction' would have made practice in sports problematic.[83] The sheer impropriety of female masseurs at the track or field would largely have prevented their engaging with sport. Thus sportsmen, presuming they had no active

injury already under medical care, would have recourse only to male masseurs, either trained but outside the Society of Trained Masseuses, or the
experienced 'rubber'.

A second barrier was the Society of Trained Masseuses's rule that
members could only advertise their services in 'strictly medical papers'.[84]
While a sportsman could, of course, buy copies of the *Medical Magazine*
or the *British Medical Journal*, it is considerably more likely that he would
apply to those masseurs advertising in the *Athletic News* or the back pages
of training manuals. Such masseurs would be outside the newly professionalised activity of massage, but this does not mean that they were in
any way *amateurs*. Training courses in massage including basic physiology and anatomy were available, at a price, to all comers.[85] So what were
the masseurs employed by athletes? Were they 'rubbers' or medically
educated masseurs? The answer is apparently both: but what is interesting is the repeated use of massage as a signal of modern, 'scientific'
training practice. Of course, *immoderate* use of massage was disparaged,
as was *immoderate* use of massage oils (particularly by foreign teams).[86]
Nonetheless the reactions of the 'old school' of coaches and trainers were
used in some sporting literature as evidence for the credentials of scientific massage. One particular story, told twice in the pages of the *Athletic
News* in 1913 and 1914, involved the coach Jack Hepplethwaite. In 1913
the cycling correspondent 'Strephon' wrote:

> I shall never forget the look on poor old Jack Hepplethwaite's face the first
> time he saw Jack Donaldson going through the mill on a table in Fallowfield,
> 'Murder!' That's what it is 'Murder!' and yet Donaldson and all the greatest
> runners of the day . . . are great believers in massage.[87]

Jack Donaldson (1886–1933) was a successful (Australian-born) professional runner; the implication that runners/athletes themselves might
have faith in a treatment that their coaches distrusted is interesting. The
masseur himself, Mr Montague Laughton, was described as a 'most
experienced masseur' and though his professional qualifications (if any)
were not mentioned he was clearly not to be considered by readers of the
*Athletic News* as 'just' a rubber.

Again, in 1914 Strephon used Hepplethwaite as an avatar of old-
fashioned coaches due to his reaction to scientific massage:

> I can remember him saying to me in the vernacular which I shall not
> attempt to commit to print – 'You're surely not going to stand by and allow
> him to rub all the good out of the lad's legs? His legs don't need massaging;
> they're clean enough; give them a wipe down; give his body a better rub and
> he'll do.'

How old Jack groused when the masseur had his way. 'Good will not come
of it,' he declared. 'Mark my words.' And I am afraid we did mark his words,
though we did not attribute consequences which shall not be mentioned here
to massage.[88]

It is worth pointing out here that although the race did not turn out in
favour of the massaged athlete, the massage treatment is not blamed (by
the author) for a poor performance. The 'traditional' amateur reliance on
the tried-and-tested mechanism did not always apply.[89]

Debates over massage in sport, how much and when it should be used,
how vigorous it should be, and what oils (if any) should be used, largely
mirrored the debates over massage in all other areas of treatment and
rehabilitation. Throughout these debates it was the *rubber* who was backwards, and the *masseur* who was scientific. Vegetarian athlete Emil Voigt
went so far, in 1914, as to compare the backwardness of 'the opponents
of scientific massage' with 'the flat-earthers' and the 'geocentricians'.[90]
Furthermore:

[t]he claims that massage is a valuable aid to training does not rest solely
upon its wide adoption by the world's best athletes, nor upon the improvement in athletic ability that followed its use ... [but] lies in its complete
accordance with the teachings of anatomy and physiology. In short, massage
works scientifically along natural lines.[91]

Massage is explicitly not 'the haphazard movements of the 'rubber' so
well known in athletic circles in England; it is the skilful manipulation of
one who is aware of the function and structure of each muscle which he
handles'.[92] Massage is also not just a training technique, it is a medical
intervention clearly grounded in contemporary physiological and clinical
thought. It is not something whose practice is a function of experience,
but is a professional activity. Here is a clear case of sports medicine in the
early twentieth century, acknowledged as such by medics and sporting
professionals alike.

J Ker Lindsay's columns of medical advice for sportsmen contained
regular references to the use of massage as a curative and restorative, since
it was 'a scientific method of treating diseases and injuries by systematic
manipulations'.[93] In 1908 Lindsay dedicated three whole articles to the
use of massage in sport. Massage also appeared at the most elite levels of
sporting activity; at the first modern Olympic Games the American high
jumpers appear to have sought the services of a masseur in the middle
of their contest. At the 1900 Paris Games, it was the (male) masseur
attached to the doctor in charge of the Gymnastic events whose services
were most in demand.[94] Masseurs and masseuses are listed as attendees

at subsequent games; certainly by 1928 some British teams were taking their own.[95]

There is little doubt that the opening of the professional certificate of massage to men and the rising numbers of those trained in massage due to the medical demands of war increased its use in the sporting world.[96] By the time Romer published his article on sporting injuries in 1923, his instruction to seek the 'services of a skilled masseur' was a common form of advice given in training manuals and medical texts.[97] Use of professional, chartered and certificated massage and physiotherapy services became standard in professional and amateur sports clubs in the 1930s and 1940s, with training schemes for coaches and trainers.[98] Such massage could be as 'scientific', or as firmly based on contemporary anatomical and physiological teaching, as that provided by certified masseuses from the Society of Trained Masseuses; it was an artefact of gender and of rules of advertising that prevented athletes from utilising the only certified masseurs of the early twentieth century. This does not imply that athletes were not interested in 'scientific' massage.

Whatever the appeal of tried-and-trusted methodology, it was clearly still possible for sports doctors to appeal to modernity in their methods. The evidence of the use (and debates over) exercise and massage in the treatment of orthopaedic injuries in sports and the preparation of athletes shows a practice essentially in sync with any other forms of 'mainstream' medicine. Self-styled modernists advised movement as life, while traditionalists acted to place checks and limits on the degree of exercise invoked (as well as criticising other 'faddy' alternatives to rest). Massage, although variously applied and interpreted, was modern – 'rubbing' old-fashioned and to be phased out. The absence of organisations, institutions, or self-identifying professionals did not mean that sports medicine was exempted from medical 'progress', nor that it created an isolated medical paradigm, distinct from non-sports medicine and health care. What it consisted of was an intricate network of enthusiasts and semi-specialists, some medically trained, some amateurs, who participated in and created a network of health beliefs; some of these had long, traditional roots, while others were interpretations of cutting edge medical research.

The emetic recipe quoted at the beginning of this chapter comes from a text which is a particularly good example of the ambiguous nature of sports medicine. It was written by the famous trainer Sam Mussabini (who coached, among others, Harold Abrahams to victory in the 100m at the 1912 Olympics), who has been characterised by other sports historians as the 'last of the old school', promoting a purgative regime for athletes, and suggesting that the skin was an organ of respiration. Yet at the same time his training manuals embrace the theories of moderation and individualism; he promoted light exercise in preference to rest as a cure for sprains and strains; he used contemporary physiological theory to analyse athletic movements; and he recommend that athletes should consult a doctor before, and during, a new training regime.[99] Therefore both contradictory characterisations – last of the old school and eager proponent of new biomedical ideas – are correct.

## Conclusion: moderate individuals

Much of this chapter has concentrated on direct treatment in sports medicine. The examples given here – diet, massage and movement, among other things – are all intended to make the point that sports medicine was neither retarded nor isolated, and athletes had access to advice and treatment on a par with their peers. In some cases they were early adopters of treatments which only later became mainstream. But this does not really demonstrate that sports medicine actually existed; it could certainly be argued that all I have done here is talk about the history of medicine applied to sport in the early twentieth century, without making the argument that this is conceptually different enough in the case of athletes to warrant a whole chapter in a book ostensibly about the history of sports medicine.

My argument is that the athlete was normal; consequently sports medicine is usually invisible. But it is not always indistinguishable. Aside from the obvious cases such as specialist knee surgeons, special diets and special hospitals, it is in the area of prevention – usually policing – that sports medicine is immediately visible even at the beginning of the twentieth century. Those sports which seemed particularly dangerous found themselves under medical control and supervision; those bodies particularly unfitted for sport were screened, examined and even forbidden from taking part.

Unsurprisingly, perhaps, it was the challenging endurance sports which first attracted medical control; cycling, rowing and the marathon. As already noted above, at the first London Olympics in 1908 medical certificates were required of all competitors in the marathon, and all had to agree to 'at once retire from the race if ordered to do so by a member of the medical staff appointed by the British Olympic Council to patrol the course'.[100] Interestingly, these games also saw the introduction of the first doping regulations, 'No competitor either at the start or during the progress of the race may take or receive any drug. The breach of this rule will operate as an absolute disqualification'.[101] This may be partly to do with the experience of the 1904 Games where the 'winning' competitor turned out to have ridden much of the course in a car, and the second-placed runner 'was running the last ounces of strength out of his body, kept in mechanical action by the use of drugs', which included strychnine, alcohol (brandy) and egg white.[102] Lurid reports of this marathon had horrified audiences:

> His eyes were dull, lusterless; the ashen color of his face and skin had deepened; his arms appeared as weights well tied down; he could scarcely lift his legs, while his knees were almost stiff. The brain was fairly normal, but there was more or less hallucination.[103]

The other area in which sports medicine used its policing remit was in the context of school games. Many doctors involved in sport fiercely disputed the suggestion that sports could be harmful for children, so the subject of vulnerable boys' bodies gradually shaded into issues of screening and policing (see Lauder Brunton's quote above: 'I am anxious not to prevent [sports] but to regulate them').[104] Cross-country running could not harm a normal healthy boy; on the other hand, it could be harmful to one whose body was unnaturally weakened by disability or hereditary infirmity, or to one who did not have the moral courage to stop when he was beaten. We must not miss what is being implied here: doctors and medical professionals are expressing authority over the athletic body by *identifying who ought or ought not to participate in sports*. While they may not yet have control of the normal athletic body, the pathological or *potentially* pathological athletic body is clearly their domain.

This tells us something quite important about the athletic body, the subject and object of sports medicine, and allow us to answer the question 'what or *who* was an athlete?' Despite suggestions that the professional sportsman was a 'rarity' and discussions of 'muscle bound freaks' and pallid vegetarian cyclists, the athletic body in the early twentieth century is the archetype of the *normal* body. Such a claim is evidenced by statements about the fringes of athletic activity, by the application of individualism and moderation, and by the evolution of screening. For the first; there *are* abnormal athletes, but the moderate athlete is the very embodiment of balanced, rational (in the scientific and moral sense) masculine health. The professional footballer may be a 'curiosity', but he is so in a cultural sense; physiologically he differs little from any other manual labourer or skilled craftsman.[105] Secondly, individualism and moderation were rules for everyone, in all walks of life, not just the sportsman and not just on the field.

Finally, there is screening; in the early twentieth century this was not employed to pick out the *best* and the few (i.e. elite Olympic athletes), but rather to weed out the *weak* and the few. In a system perhaps influenced by screening for warfare, where necessity dictates that most should pass, cross-country was suitable for all but the sickliest boys, the marathon for all healthy young men. While biomedical principles were included and absorbed into early twentieth-century enhancement practices, it was most specifically the pathological athletic body (or would-be athletic body) over which the doctor had dominion; the injured athlete, or the civilian predisposed to heart disease. The athletic body was normal, and it could not be hurt or harmed by 'normal' athletic activity; it was only abnormal (immoderate) activity which had to be refrained from entirely, and, vice versa, only abnormal bodies which had to refrain from normal activity.

While the athlete as normal, avatar, and archetype is a persistent symbol, the next 25 years of the twentieth century resulted in the formation of a professionalised group of sports medics. To sustain a separate identity these men needed to construct a clear and distinct patient group. Although activity and location still played a role, the athletic body also underwent a redefinition, shifting (or being shifted by) the nature and practice of sports medicine in Britain. It is these changes which are discussed in the next chapter.

## Notes

1 Recipe for a purgative to cleanse the stomach and liver before starting a training regime for sprint running. SA Mussabini, *The Complete Athletic Coach* (Methuen & Co. Ltd: London, 1913), p. 27.
2 Although it is harder to find, there is also some evidence that athletes themselves actively sought out 'scientific' advice and training methods; at least, they certainly complained when they did not get them. See for example James Lawrence 'the famous international' Association Footballer complaining that in the early twentieth century 'not enough attention was given to putting a player's preparation on sound, scientific lines'. J Lawrence, 'A Goalkeeper's Life Story' *Athletic News*, 30 May 1921.
3 See: JA Mangan, *Athleticism in the Victorian and Edwardian Public School* (Cambridge: Cambridge University Press, 1981).
4 Probably the first was: FA Schmidt and EH Miles, The Training of the Body for Games, Athletics, Gymnastics and Other Forms of Exercise and for Health, Growth and Development (New York; London: S. Sonnenschein & Company / EP Dutton & Co, 1901).
5 John Rylands University Library of Manchester, Special Collections: ARC 4/6 Log Books 1906–8.
6 E Toon and J Golden, "Live Clean, Think Clean, and Don't go to Burlesque Shows': Charles Atlas as Health Advisor' *Journal of the History of Medicine and Allied Sciences* 57 (2002), 39–60; DL Chapman, *Sandow the Magnificent: Eugen Sandow and the Beginnings of Bodybuilding* (Urbana: University of Illinois Press, 1994).

7  Although slightly without the chronology of this chapter, a particularly good example of the division between an 'athlete' and an (unhealthy) muscular type see this ongoing debate in the *Lancet*: J Plesch, 'Arterial Atony and Arterio-Sclerosis' *Lancet* 219 (1932), 385–91; A Abrahams, 'Arterial Atony and Arterio-Sclerosis' *Lancet* 219 (1932), 480; J Plesch, 'Arterial Atony and Arterio-Sclerosis' *Lancet* 219 (1932), 641–2; A Abrahams, 'Arterial Atony and Arterio-Sclerosis' *Lancet* 219 (1932), 700.

8  Anon, 'Athleticism – mens sana – the Cult of Muscle' *Manchester Guardian*, 17 June 1904.

9  V Heggie, 'A Century of Cardiomythology: Exercise and the Heart c1880–1980' *Social History of Medicine* 23 (2010), 280–98. See also C Lawrence, 'Moderns and Ancients: the 'New Cardiology' in Britain 1880–1930' *Medical History* 5 (1985), 1–33; JD Howell, '"Soldier's Heart": The Redefinition of Heart Disease and Specialty Formation in Early Twentieth-Century Great Britain' *Medical History* 5 (1985), 34–52; JC Whorton, ''Athlete's Heart': The Medical Debate Over Athleticism, 1870–1920' *Journal of Sport History* 9 (1982), 30–52.

10 R Beamish and I Ritchie, 'From Fixed Capacities to Performance-Enhancement: The Paradigm Shift in the Science of "Training" and the Use of Performance-Enhancing Substances' *Sport in History* 25 (2005), 412-33; RJ Park, 'Athletes and Their Training in Britain and America' in J Berryman & R Park (eds) *Sport and Exercise Science: Essays in the History of Sports Medicine* (Chicago: University of Illinois Press, 1992), 57–107.

11 Anon, 'En Passant: A Mishap at Liverpool' *Athletic News*, 30 Sep. 1907.

12 See also the specialist treatment described in Anon, 'En Passant: Serious accident to A Ducat' *Athletic News*, 16 Sep. 1912.

13 On the traditional chronology see R Holt and T Mason, *Sport in Britain, 1945–2000* (Oxford: Blackwell, 2000).

14 *Athletic News*, 3 July 1905.

15 Centre for Sports Science & History, Birmingham University [Hence: CSSH] Archives of the Amateur Athletics Association. AAA/3/7/2, *Scrapbook of the 1908 Olympics*.

16 British Olympic Council, *The Fourth Olympiad: London 1908* (London: British Olympic Council, 1908), pp. 71.

17 Ibid.

18 Anon, 'New Mills and Newtown, Capital Racing but poor sport' *Athletic News*, 13 July 1914.

19 Just as examples: the rugby player AH Hornby consulted a 'Harley-street specialist' about his abdominal strain in 1907, and the Association Footballer Samuel Wightman's fatal burst intestine was treated 'by a London specialist' (to no avail). Such treatment was not limited to London or Harley Street, because, also in 1912, Tottenham Hotspur's player Walkden visited 'at least two specialists' about his knee injury 'making one journey to the North of England to secure advice'. Anon, 'En Passant: AH Hornby's Accident' *Athletic News*, 20 May 1907; Anon, 'En Passant: Death of a Full Back' *Athletic News* 15 Apr. 1912.

20 Anon, 'En Passant: the Case of Frank Ward' *Athletic News*, 28 June 1909.
21 Anon, 'The Olympic Games – chances of the English Men' *Athletic News*, 16 Apr. 1906.
22 B Mallon and I Buchanan, *The 1908 Olympic Games: Results for All Competitors in All events, with commentary* (North Carolina; London: McFarland and Company, 2000), p. 7.
23 Ibid., pp. 72, 410. Rapports – Exposition Universelle International de 1900 á Paris [Including the Official Report of the Olympic Games] (Paris: Ministére Du Commerce, De L'Industrie des Postes et des Télégraphes, 1900).
24 British Olympic Council, *The Fourth Olympiad: London 1908* , pp. 78.
25 As quoted in Mallon and Buchanan, *The 1908 Olympic Games*, p. 324.
26 Ibid., p. 142.
27 BOC, *The Fourth Olympiad: London 1908*, p. 695.
28 The Official Report notes just 149 'cases' treated in the stadium (including 17 women); these ranged from bruises and grazes, through tonsillitis and broken ribs (as well as one 'wound caused by a hat-pin' in a female gymnast). Stockholm Organising Committee, *The Olympic Games of Stockholm 1912* (Stockhom: Swedish Olympic Committee/Wahlstrom & Widstrand, 1912). Tables I – IV.
29 Ibid., p. 839.
30 Unless otherwise stated details come from the official report, *The Olympic Games of Stockholm 1912.*
31 'Il sera nécessaire en tous cas que désormais la course de Marathon soit placée dans la matinée et surtout que des mesures sévères soient prises pour empêcher les concurrents d'absorber en cours de route des aliments nocifs' Anon, 'Une Olympiade à vol doiseau' [In the future the Marathon race should be scheduled for the morning, and serious measures should be taken to prevent the competitors from taking harmful substances/foodstuffs during the course of the race.] *Revue Olympique* 80 (1912), 115–99. 118.
32 A Rabinbach, *The Human Motor: Energy, Fatigue and the Origins of Modernity* (California: University of California Press, 1992).
33 On the importance of the moral component of physical activity see: N Garnham, 'Both Praying and Playing: 'Muscular Christianity' and the YMCA in north-east County Durham' *Journal of Social History* 35 (2) 2001, 397–407; Mangan, *Athleticism*; JA Mangan, '"Muscular, Militaristic and Manly": The British Middle-class Hero as Moral Messenger' *International Journal of the History of Sport* 13 (1996), 28–47.
34 For an example applied to diet, see: A Abrahams, 'The Scientific Side of Athletics', in EH Ryle and EE White (eds), *Athletics (The National Library of Sports and Pastimes)* (London: Eveleigh Nash, 1912), pp. 29–40. 40.
35 [CSSH] II.A696, Sprinter, 'Hints on Diet' in 'Sprinter' (ed.), *The Athletic News Handbook on Training for Athletes and Cyclists* (c. 1902), p. 6.
36 Abrahams, 'The Scientific Side', pp. 41–2.
37 J Ker Lindsay, 'Medical Miscellany – Does Exercise Shorten Life?' *Athletic News*, 3 Feb. 1908. See below for more on Ker Lindsay and his medical columns.

38 It also applied to smoking: 'the weight of evidence is in favour of the view that tobacco smoked in moderation by full-grown healthy adults is not injurious to the system.' J Ker Lindsay, 'Medical Miscellany – Use and abuse of tobacco' *Athletic News*, 10 Feb. 1908.

39 RJ Park, '"Mended or Ended?": Football Injuries and the British and American Medical Press, 1870–1910' *The International Journal of the History of Sport* 18 (June 2001), 110–33.

40 Anon, 'Wheel World' *Athletic News*, 28 Dec. 1908.

41 'A Practicing Physician', 'Healthy Exercise, The Dangers Of Systems' *Athletic News*, 18 Apr. 1910.

42 Including Emil Voigt, the Manchester-born runner who took gold in the Five Mile Race at the 1908 London Olympics; Voigt was a dedicated vegetarian, although he chose the lifestyle due to ethical rather than health concerns. Anon, 'The Olympic Games: World's Athletes At The Stadium – Linguist, Vegetarian, Champion – the Life Story of Emil Voigt' *Athletic News*, 20 Jul. 1908.

43 V Heggie, 'Lies, Damn Lies and Manchester's Recruiting Statistics: Degeneration as an "Urban Legend" in Victorian and Edwardian Britain' *Journal of the History of Medicine and Allied Sciences*, 63 (2008), 178–216.

44 Notions of physical degeneration and accompanying physical stigmata also played a role – for this see D Pick, *Faces of Degeneration: A European disorder c1848–1918* (Cambridge: Cambridge University Press, 1989).

45 S West, 'Heart Strain, with Some Remarks on Training and Other Allied Cardiac Conditions' *Practitioner* 2 (1911), 137–46. 139.

46 Reported in: W Collier, *School Athletics and Boys' Races* (London: J&A Churchill, 1909), p. 14.

47 Ibid.

48 M Randal Roberts, 'A Footballers' Hospital' *The Windsor Magazine* (March 1899), 511–16.

49 A Abrahams, 'Athletics and the Medical Man' *Practitioner* 86 (1911), 429–46. 430.

50 The letter forwarded to the *Times* was signed by only five (not the six that Abrahams claims) doctors, Sir Lauder Brunton (1844–1916), Sir Thomas Barlow (1845–1945), Sir James F. Goodhart (1845–1916), Sir William Hale-White (1857–1949), and Sir Alfred Fripp (1865–1930). All of these men were nationally recognised medics and surgeons, and the latter was surgeon to the King. 'Letter: Boys' Races' *Times*, 8 Feb. 1909.

51 W Collier, *School Athletics*; 'Notes By The Way: Races for Boys' *The Practitioner* 1 (1909), 572–3; 'Boys' Races' *Times*, 8, 9, 10, 12, 15, 16, 17, 19 Feb. and 12 Mar. 1909.

52 '[F]ormerly Scholar of Kings College Cambridge, Member of the Executive Council of the National League of Physical Education and Improvement, Amateur Champion of England at Tennis, 1899 to 1903, 1905, 1906, 1909, 1910, and at Racquets, 1902 and in the doubles 1902, 1904 to 1906 of America at Racquets, Tennis, and Squash – Tennis, 1900, Holder of the Gold Prize'. E

Miles, *Restaurant Recipes* (Eustace Miles: London, 1906); Miles with Schmidt, *The Training of the Body*. Criticised as a faddist for his '"rissoles with curry flavour," his "rice cutlets," and his "vegetable roast"' in 'Notes by the Way: Food Fads' *The Practitioner* 1 (1905), 852.

53 'Had an English cook been carried on that expedition [to the 1912 Olympiad], and had such plain food been prepared as the athletes were accustomed to, the expense would have been justified'. Anon, 'Topics of the Track' *Athletic News*, 28. June 1915.

54 RJ Park, 'High-Protein Diets, 'Damaged Hearts', and Rowing Men: Antecedents of Modern Sports Medicine and Exercise Science, 1867–1928', *Exercise and Sports Science Reviews* 25 (1997), 137–69. 147.

55 CH Larette, 'How to Get Fit and Keep So' in 'Sprinter' (ed.) *The Athletic News Handbook on Training for Athletes and Cyclists* (London: Athletic News *c*. 1902), p. 48.

56 W Thom, Pedestrianism, or, An Account of the Performances of Celebrated Pedestrians During the Last and Present Century (Aberdeen: D Chalmers & Co, 1812), pp. 232–5.

57 P Mewett, 'Sports training, science and class among British amateur athletes in the mid to late nineteenth century' in J Northcote (ed.) *Sociology for a Mobile World: Conference Proceedings of The Australian Sociological Association 2006 Conference*, (Australia: The Sociological Association of Australia, 2006), pp. 1–10.

58 This is an ongoing controversy: MW Cooke, *et al*, 'A survey of current consultant practice of treatment of severe ankle sprains in emergency departments in the United Kingdom' *Emergency Medicine Journal* 20 (2003), 505–7; C Zöch, V Fialka-Moser, M Quittan, 'Rehabilitation of ligamentous ankle injuries: a review of recent studies' *BJSM* 37 (2003), 291–5.

59 J Hilton, *On Rest and Pain* (London: JG Bell & Sons, 1877).

60 J Barclay, *In Good Hands: The History of the Chartered Society of Physiotherapy 1894–1994* (London: Butterworth-Heinemann, 1994), p. 17. The original French text came out in 1885: J Lucas-Championère, *Traitement des fractures par le massage et la mobilisation* (Paris, 1885). See also a positive English-language review – FC Husson, 'Lucas Championnere on Massage and Mobilisation in the Treatment of Fractures' *Annals of Surgery* 11 (1889), 359–64.

61 Bennett was an eminent British surgeon based at St Guy's Hospital, London. WH Bennett, 'On the Use of Massage in The treatment of Recent Fractures' *Lancet* 151 (1898), 359–61. 360.

62 WH Bennett, 'The Use of Massage in Recent Fractures and Other Common Injuries' *Lancet* 155 (1900), 1569–74, 1640–3. 1640.

63 O Holst, 'Letter: Massage and Movement in Sprains and Dislocations' *Lancet* 160 (1902), 1424–5. 1425.

64 R Warren, 'The Fate of Damaged Joints: a study of cases of injury, principally fractures, involving joints treated in the massage department of the London Hospital' *Lancet* 174 (1909), 219–22. 222.

65  JB Mennell, 'The Treatment of Recent Injury by Mobilisation and Massage' *Lancet* 181 (1913), 316–17. 316.

66  Ibid.

67  R Cooter, 'The Meaning of Fractures: Orthopaedics and the Reform of British Hospitals in the Inter-war Period' *Medical History* 31 (1987), 306–32.

68  After the treatment became almost universally recommended by articles and textbooks in the 1930s and 1940s, training and sports medicine handbooks instead sometimes blamed athletes for being ignorant about sprains, and for tending to rest rather than exercise. See WE Tucker, 'Fitness and Training' in JR Armstrong & WE Tucker (eds), *Injury in Sport – The Physiology, Prevention and treatment of Injuries associated with Sport* (London: Staples Press, 1964), pp. 82–93.

69  Rex Salisbury Woods (1892–1986) was a Cambridge doctor, and shot-put competitor for Britain in the 1924 and 1928 Games. 'He . . . specialis[ed] in the treatment of athletes long before there were any official sports medicine organisations', and was a founder (and later life) member of BAS(E)M. RS Woods, 'Beating the Clock: Evolution in the Treatment of Sports Injuries' *Practitioner* 203 (1969), 329–36. 329; Anon, 'News of Members' *BJSM*, 15 (1981), 220; HE Robson, 'Obituary: Rex Salisbury Woods' *BJSM*, 20 (1986), 187.

70  Woods, 'Beating the Clock', 329.

71  F Romer, 'Sports Injuries' *Practitioner*, 1 (1923), 99–112.

72  J Ker Lindsay, 'Medical Miscellany – Sprains of the Knee Joint ' *Athletic News*, 21 Oct. 1907.

73  J Ker Lindsay, 'Medical Miscellany – Injuries to the Ankle Joint' *Athletic News*, 14 Oct. 1907.

74  J Ker Lindsay, 'Medical Miscellany' *Athletic News*, 16 Nov. 1908.

75  'APP', 'Neglected Sprains – Danger of Developments' *Athletic News*, 24 Apr. 1910.

76  Roberts, 'A Footballers' Hospital'.

77  N Carter, 'The Rise and Fall of the Magic Sponge: Football Trainers and the Persistence of Popular Medicine' *Social History of Medicine* 23 (2010), 261–79, 274.

78  The Society of Trained Masseuses merged with the Manchester-based Institute of Massage and Remedial Gymnastics in 1920, becoming the Chartered Society of Massage and Medical Gymnastics. It was renamed as the Chartered Society of Physiotherapy in 1943. Jean Barclay, *In Good Hands*, pp. 70, 125.

79  For the scandal's impact on massage and physiotherapy as professions see DA Nicholls and J Cheek, 'The Society of Trained Masseuses and the massage scandals of 1894' *Social Science and Medicine* 62 (2006), 236–48. For contemporary commentary see: Anon, 'The Scandals of Massage: Report of the Special Commissioners of the 'British Medical Journal' *BMJ* 1 (1894), 1003–4; Anon, 'The Medical Profession and Massage Establishments' *Lancet*

149 (1897), 538; Anon, 'The Medical Profession and Massage Establishments' *Lancet* 152 (1898), 1073; Anon, 'The Massage Scandals' *Lancet* 153 (1899), 1310–11.

80 JH Wickstead, *The Growth of A Profession, being the history of the Chartered Society of Physiotherapy, 1894–1945* (London: Edward Arnold & Co, 1948). See also Chapter 6 'The Great War' in R Cooter, *Surgery and Society in Peace and War: Orthopaedics and the Organisation of Modern Medicine, 1880–1948* (London: Macmillan, 1993).

81 '[T]he 'rubber,' [was] a man who massaged athletes before and after competition, applied such taping as was used, acted as first-aid man in a very crude fashion . . . [he] was usually a man without formal education beyond high school, often a former athlete, who worked by tradition, favored home remedies, and generally ignored advice.' AJ Ryan, *Medical Care of the Athlete* (London; New York; Toronto: McGraw-Hill, 1963), pp. 49–50.

82 The only eligible men were army orderlies and asylum attendants. This remained the case until 1915 when the Institute of Massage and Remedial Gymnastics was formed in Manchester; the two organisations amalgamated in 1920, opening membership of the joint society to men and women. Barclay, *In Good Hands*. Many training institutions, however, remained female only: John Rylands University of Manchester. Manchester Medical Collection. MMC/9/6/15/4/1. *Prospectus of the School of Massage*. See footnote 85, below.

83 Barclay, *In Good Hands*, pp. 26–7.

84 Ibid., p. 27.

85 Including those women trained in massage through their work in remedial gymnastics, and men and women with visual impairments trained by the Institute for Massage by the Blind founded in 1900. Anon, 'Orthodox Medical Gymnastics and Medical Massage' *Lancet* 166 (1905), 1570; Anon, 'Massage by the Blind' *Lancet* 168 (1906), 1527–8.

86 According to the *Athletic News'* cycling correspondent, 'Yankee athletes simply revelled in massage. Their army of rubbers were kept busy, and [their changing tent for the 1908 Olympic Games] reeked of witch hazel, wintergreen, heartshorn, eucalyptus and such things'. 'Strephon', 'Topics of the Track' *Athletic News*, 1 June 1914.

87 'Strephon', 'Topics of the Track' *Athletic News*, 20 May 1913.

88 'Strephon', 'Topics of the Track' *Athletic News*, 1 June 1914.

89 The use of 'science' to differentiate between the new middle-class athlete and the working-class professional coach is explored above.

90 Anon, 'Massage treatment – Its Value to Athletes' *Athletic News*, 20 July 1914.

91 Ibid.

92 J Ker Lindsay, 'Medical Miscellany – Stages of Massage' *Athletic News*, 24 Feb. 1908.

93 Ibid.

94 'Nous devons ajouter qu'un masseur avait été spéclialement attaché au docteur et que c'est lui qui a eu á faire la plus grande partied du travail.'

Rapports – Exposition Universelle International de 1900 á Paris [Including the Official Report of the Olympic Games] (Paris: Ministére Du Commerce, De L'Industrie des Postes et des Télégraphes, 1900), p. 119.

95 Netherlands Olympic Committee, *The Ninth Olympiad – Official Report* (Netherlands: Netherlands Olympic Committee, 1928).

96 The membership of the Incorporated Society of Trained Masseuses numbered around 200 in 1900, and by 1918 membership could be measured in the thousands. MV Lace, *Massage and Medical Gymnastics* (London: J&A Churchill Ltd, 1945), p. 3.

97 See, for example, H Andrews, *Training for the Track, Field, and Road with some hints on Health and Fitness* (London: Stanley Paul, 1914), written by a professional trainer for an amateur athletic audience; this heavily emphasises and promotes the value of 'scientific massage', and the vital importance of securing a 'professional' masseur to deliver it.

98 N Carter, 'Metatarsals and Magic Sponges: English Football and the Development of Sports Medicine' *Journal of Sport History* 34 (2007), 53–74.

99 McNab *et al.* in *The UK Literature of Track and Field* (2001) state that 'the reader of the Complete Athletic Coach will occasionally find statements which might well have been penned by Captain Barclay over a century before'. Compare this to Terry's assertion (2000) that 'Mussabini started applying new technology to his training methods . . . [the Complete Coach] describes advanced methods of training and technique from the sprints to the marathon'. T McNab, P Lovesey, A Huxtable, *The UK Literature of Track and Field* (London: British Library, 2001); D Terry, 'An Athletic Coach Ahead of his Time' *British Society of Sports History Newsletter* 11 (Spring 2000), 34–8; S Mussabini, *Track and Field Athletics: A Guide to Correct Training* (Foulsham: London, 1924); Mussabini, *The Complete Athletic Coach*.

100 The Fourth Olympiad: London 1908, p. 88.

101 Ibid.

102 CJP Lucas, *The Olympic Games 1904* (St Louis: Woodward & Tiernan, 1905), p. 53.

103 Ibid.

104 Collier, *School Athletics*, p. 14.

105 This was reflected in the application of the National Insurance Act of 1911 and the Workman's Compensation Act of 1906, which were applied to professional footballers (after some legal wrangling). *Athletic News*, 17 Jun. 1912.

### Box 1. The Footballers' Hospital

Matlock House, also known as the 'Footballers' Hospital', was owned by John Allison (*c.*1850–1919) – see also Figure 2. Originally an institute for general hydrotherapy, endowed by a legacy from a successfully treated 'Bolton millionaire and MP', the hospital gradually became popular with sportsmen, particularly professional footballers.[1] Allison himself expressed his own interest in sport by becoming involved in the management/committee work of Old Ardwick and Manchester City Football Clubs, as well as being the president of the local Salford Harriers Athletic Club. The hospital was founded in the late 1870s, and moved to its Hyde Road location in the early 1880s. As well as the hydrotherapy indicated in the hospital's name, it also offered heat-treatment 'applying a tremendous heat by means of electricity...It is essentially a dry heat, and . . . a temperature of no less than 500 degrees can be endured without discomfort' and other associated therapies.[2]

Allison also offered treatment 'on the pitch' to players, as well as detecting those faking injuries with a terrifying 'sham detector', consisting of a plaster and a poultice of secret ingredients, whose 'chief virtue [was] that it [was] diabolically painful as well as lasting in its effects.'[2] It appears that the driving force behind the specialism of the hospital was Allison himself, since by 1925, six years after his death, the institution had been taken over by the local authorities and seemed to lose its special interest in sports injuries.

[1] I Nannestad, 'John Allison and his Football hospital' *Soccer History* 9 (Autumn 2004), 42–3.

[2] M Randal Roberts, 'A Footballers' Hospital' *The Windsor Magazine* (March 1899), 511–16.

---

*Box 2. Adolphe Abrahams (1883–1967)*

Dr Adolphe Abrahams, OBE, MD, FRCP, was one of Britain's foremost sports medics; founder of several organisations dedicated to sports medicine, and publisher of a host of books, articles and monographs relating to sports medicine and sports science. Elder brother of the more athletically talented Harold Abrahams (sprinter), he attended several Olympic Games in a medical capacity; travelling with the Athletics team in 1908 and 1912, and more formally as an Honorary Medical Officer for the BOA from 1924 onwards.[1,2] Adolphe claimed to have also attended the 1904 games.[3]

A keen sportsman, Abrahams served in the Royal Army Medical Corps between 1915 and 1920, before getting a civilian job at the Westminster Hospital.[1] In 1951 he was involved in the formation of an Athlete's Advisory Committee for the Amateur Athletics Association, and in 1952 collaborated with Sir Arthur Porritt in the founding of the British Association of Sport and Medicine, becoming its first President (until his death in 1967). Abrahams was also the chairman of the Medical Committee of the National Fitness Council, (1937–39).

Although advocating a more scientific approach to training and competition, Abrahams also strongly promoted a 'for the love of the game' ethic in sport, decrying what he saw as the 'preposterous standard' of the modern Olympic Games which had 'perverted and distorted the original idea of recreative and competitive athletics by demanding the production of the super-athlete.'[4]

[1] 'Sir Adolphe Abrahams' *Times*, 12 Dec. 1967. (Obituary).
[2] Details taken from the various British Olympic Association Team Handbooks.
[3] Adolphe Abrahams, 'Athletic Training: The Olympic Standard' *Times*, 4 Aug. 1931.
[4] Adolphe Abrahams, *The Disabilities and Injuries of Sport* (London: Elek Books Ltd, 1961).
See also: LA Reynolds & EM Tansey (eds), *The Development of Sports Medicine in Twentieth Century Britain* (London: Wellcome Trust, 2009), p. 113.

## Box 3. *Staleness*

Staleness is a 'bogey' which has haunted athletes throughout the twentieth century. Like the Athlete's Heart, its causes and cures have varied widely, but its symptoms remained constant. The early signs of staleness were 'early fatigue, insomnia and weight loss', and it could eventually lead to chronic physical and mental fatigue, precipitating an early retirement for the athlete.[1]

One constant in staleness has been the role of psychology in its cause and cure. Prior to World War I both food and 'over-training' ('to take more from [the body] than [training] puts into it') were blamed – 'care in the diet prevents staleness' wrote Adolphe Abrahams in 1912.[2,3] Yet part of the cause of staleness lay in the mind; the mental strain of over-training, or the monotony and unpleasantness of an inappropriate, non-individual, or invariable diet.

With the isolation of hormones in the 1930s and 1940s, and accompanying physiological concentration on such biochemistry, there were suggestions that staleness was caused by an accumulation of a 'fatigue toxin', or by auto-intoxication from the adrenal glands; 'its symptoms of weakness and lassitude, anorexia and weight loss, its signs of sunken eyes and flabbiness of muscle are reminiscent of chronic adrenal exhaustion.'[4,5]

Still, the mental aspect remained important. Abrahams particularly championed the psychological causes, arguing that a lack of adequate rest periods caused staleness by preventing the subconscious from having enough time to 'active[ly] prep[are] to assist the conscious when the occasion demands'.[6] The 'cure' (or preventive) for staleness in the first half of the twentieth century could therefore be stimulants, like alcohol[7], strychnine[8], or complete rest[5], never 'overtraining'[9], and even the use of 'ox-liver concentrate'.[10]

By the 1970s the psychological aspect of staleness came to the fore and the condition became closely associated with Chronic Fatigue Syndrome. As explanations for Chronic Fatigue have varied from mental illness to viral infection, so has the explanation for athletic staleness.[11] Staleness has never coalesced into a distinct clinical entity, and has therefore appeared to have a straightforward cure or preventive; this has probably added to athletes' fear of this 'bogey'.

[1] JR Armstrong and WE Tucker, *Injury in Sport – The Physiology, Prevention and Treatment of Injuries Associated with Sport* (London: Staples Press, 1964), p. 108.

[2] Harry Andrews, *Training for the Track, Field, and Road with Some Hints on Health and Fitness* (London: Stanley Paul, 1914), p. 19.

[3] Adolphe Abrahams, 'The Scientific Side of Athletics' in EH Ryle and EE White (eds), *Athletics (The National Library of Sports and Pastimes)* (London: Eveleigh Nash, 1912), 29–40. 40.

[4] [CSSH] XXV.A7. A Abrahams, *The 4th Crookes Lecture, Athletic Training Past and Present*, Issued by the Athletes Advisory Service, The Crookes Laboratories Limited, London NW10. 26 Jan. 1955.

[5] JE Lovelock, 'Physiotherapy and the Athlete' *Practitioner* **158**(1947), 226–32. 232.

[6] [CSSH] XXV.M2. A Abrahams, *The Limit of Athletic Ability*, monograph, *c*. 1953.

[7]  KS Duncan, *The Oxford Pocket Book of Athletic Training* (Oxford: Oxford University Press, 1948), p. 76.

[8]  A Abrahams, 'Athletics and the Medical Man' *Practitioner* 86(1911), 429–46. 440.

[9]  H Andrews and WS Alexander, *The Secret of Athletic Training* (London: Methuen & Co., 1925), p. 17.

[10]  C Woodard, *Sports Injuries: Prevention and Active treatment* (London: Max Parrish, 1954), p. 38.

[11]  MB Bottomley, 'The Stale Athlete' *Athletics Coach* 23(1989), 25–6.

# 3

# Ideal citizens? Research and injuries, 1928–52

The year 1928, where this chapter starts, would stand out in any sports medicine chronology.[1] In February 1928 a meeting of physicians at the Winter Olympics in St Moritz led to the foundation of the *Association Internationale Medico-Sportive* (AIMS), later to become the *Fédération Internationale de Médecine Sportive* (FIMS) in 1934.[2] In Germany, full-time chairs in Sports Medicine were founded at universities in Hamburg and Leipzig, and the first edition of the journal *Arbeitsphysiologie*, for 'scientific reports of exercise and athletics', was published.[3] In March 1928 Adolphe Abrahams addressed the Royal College of Surgeons, giving the prestigious Arris and Gale lecture on the topic of 'Physiology of Violent Exercise in Relation to Possible Strain'.[4] Also in March 1928, the *British Medical Journal* commented on the rise of professional sports medicine in Germany, noting that although:

> there have been and are in this country surgeons with special experience in the pursuit of various sports . . . no attempt has as yet been made to develop the study of these injuries into a specialty.[5]

That said, the BOA appointed its first official Medical Officer in 1928, and Abrahams (long their 'unofficial' MO) undertook a physiological survey of potential British Olympic competitors.[6] British doctors and physiologists were among those who conducted extensive tests on track athletes at the Amsterdam Games, in the summer of 1928.

This increased interest in exercise physiology had partly been stimulated by the publication in 1927 of both *Muscular Movement in Man* and *Living Machinery* by Nobel-Prize winning British physiologist, AV Hill (Box 4).[7] Significantly too, in 1931, eight years after Frank Romer's first article on sports injuries, came the first book on sports injuries – Charles Heald's *Injuries and Sport*.[8] In this period the British government also took a renewed interest in physical education and national fitness, passing the Physical Training and Recreation Act in 1937.[9] Changes in the mechanism and direction of government funding, and in the structure and practice of research in the universities led to a snowballing production of physiological knowledge about the human body at work and play. Changes in the funding and status of orthopaedics, rehabilitation and other medical disciplines also influenced research practice, and the production of specific knowledge about the injured athlete.[10]

World War II interrupted the patterns of much of this research, but it also provided a valuable opportunity for British sport (and thus sports medicine) in the form of the London Olympics of 1948, coinciding almost to the day with the introduction of a nationalised health service. Olympic medical provision had become more comprehensive in 1932 at Los Angeles with the development of the Olympic Village system; the social and financial challenges of the 'austerity games' did not allow all these new services to be mirrored in post-war London, although, as this chapter shows, the Medical Committee certainly sought to bring cutting-edge medical practice to international athletes. The chapter ends in 1952, with the formation of Britain's first sports medicine organisation – the British Association of Sport and Medicine (BAS(E)M), founded by, among others, Adolphe Abrahams and Sir Arthur Porritt (Box 5).

Clearly, this was a particularly complex and formative time in the history of sports medicine. National and global events – a war, a nationalised health service – impacted upon the structure, function and self-conceptualisation of British sport and British medicine. Yet even in this confusion there are still some patterns which can be drawn out. Of greatest significance to this account is the emergence of a professional group of specialists in sports medicine. These men came from a range of disciplines and fields – they were doctors, physiologists, orthopaedic surgeons, ex-athletes, coaches, trainers, physiotherapists. The causes of the appearance (and congregation) of these specialists were threefold. Firstly, the financial and social effects of war; the soldier's body bears much similarity to the athlete's body, and the resulting investment in some medical disciplines (e.g. orthopaedics, rehabilitation) had a constructive effect on sports medicine, almost as a side-effect.[11] This impact was not just financial – the shifting focus of medicine and clinical research also resulted in a body of medics and researchers with a special interest in an unusual patient group of young, fit men. In peacetime it is practically only sport that provides a similar demographic group.

The second influence driving the formation of specialist groups was the pressure of conflict and inter-war depression, which created new concerns about the health of the nation. Rationing, the need for a substantial population of army-ready men, and the discussion and debate that prefigured the NHS, all led to an increasing interest in physical fitness. This is evidenced by the formation of organisations such as the Central Council of

Physical Recreation (CCPR: see Box 6) in 1935, and the National Fitness Council which ran from 1937–39, a consequence of the Physical Training and Recreation Act of 1937 which aimed to increase the availability of sites for exercise.[12]

Thirdly, and finally, there was international pressure. Although the zenith of 'sports as sublimated war' did not come until the 1950s, and was a reflection of Cold War politics, the 1930s and 1940s saw the first stirrings of a newly competitive international sporting scene. It was in the Olympic Games of the 1930s and 1940s that doping and gender fraud first became issues of concern.[13] As the quote from the *British Medical Journal* above suggests, in Britain there were specific worries that Germany in particular seemed to have outpaced Britain in its professionalisation of sports medicine. With hindsight we can see that, Germany aside, Britain was keeping pace with developments in sports medicine internationally. Britain's first book on sports injuries was published in 1931 – the first such in the US appeared in 1938.[14] Likewise, Britain saw the foundation of BAS(E)M in 1952, which affiliated with FIMS in 1953; the American College of Sports Medicine was not founded until the following year (1954).[15] (See Chapter 6 for a more extensive comparison between the UK and other countries.)

In this period, something is also happening to the athlete's body, in terms of how it is conceptualised and treated by the 'new' sports medicine professionals, and in turn by the public. This change is harder to pin down, as the identity of the athlete is essentially in flux. In part, athletes are (as the chapter title suggests) 'ideal citizens' – fit, healthy, unafraid of hard work, determined, courageous, dedicated, motivated.[16] Yet along-side this conceptualisation a new type of athlete was emerging; muscle bound, fixated with winning; demonstrating a physique and ability unobtainable by the majority; state-sponsored, professional or shamateur.[17] By this period it was no longer tenable, as it had been in 1908, or even 1924, that a reasonably fit adult could approach the performance of an elite-level athlete.[18] Although it took another decade for some parts of the British sporting world to admit as much, by 1952 the athletic body was in some respects no longer the avatar of healthy normality, but, rather, supernormal (or even abnormal).

This shift is partially a consequence of an emerging specialist group, as by definition a specialist group requires a specific object of study. While other medical disciplines concentrate on a tissue or disease type, body region or life stage, for sports medicine to become a specialty either the activity of sport must become a special activity, in terms of its biomedical consequences, or athletes must become different to the norm – or both. Most commonly, it was the athlete, not his sport, which became abnormal or supernormal. The first sports medicine books were in fact sports injury books; most made the point that sports injuries were not medical events unique to sports. Sprains, strains, athlete's foot and even tennis elbow were not the exclusive domain of the athlete. Instead these texts were justified firstly because there apparently existed a specific body of people, both medically trained and untrained, whose interests and activity lay in the area of sport and games. They therefore needed a textbook tailored to *their* practice – a body of specialists required specialist text.[19] Secondly, and increasingly over the time period covered in this book, the argument was made that although the injury might not be unique the requirements of an athlete as a patient were; their physique, physical demands, need to return to play, and even temperament and psychology all demanded 'special' treatment regimes.[20]

Finally, we should acknowledge the reality of international competition at this time. The greatly improved performance at the international level in virtually all sports also placed demands on the sports medicine professional, and the athletic body. To effectively compete against the full time athlete of Eastern Europe and the US, British athletes now had to train intensively, and under the guidance of experts. While there were those in sports medicine (for example, Adolphe Abrahams) who bemoaned the increasing competitiveness and standards of international sport, and feared the emergence of the 'unnatural athlete', the genuine pressure exerted by international competition required the production of an athletic body which was an exception, not the norm.[21]

### New sites for sports medicine

The idea of the athlete as an exception can be seen in all areas of sports medical practice; treatment, enhancement and policing. The medical supervision of sports regarded as dangerous and/or morally suspect (virtually all women's events, boxing, the marathon, and so on) continued or increased, but it was not until the athletic body, in this period acknowledged as different, began to be more specifically defined in the 1950s and 1960s that policing became the single most expensive and internationally contentious issue in sports medicine. Consequently much sports medicine practice was still concerned with the treatment of injuries and rehabilitation, or with basic studies of fitness; in both these areas the rationale for certain treatments was increasingly based on the principle that the athlete was different – either physiologically different, or socially different (i.e. requiring more active rehabilitation processes, or a more complete return to function). Auxiliary services provided to athletes increased – the number of official medical professionals travelling with the British Olympic team rose from one in 1928 (with the women's swimming team) to eight masseurs, two physiotherapists and an extra Medical Officer at the 1948 Games in London.[22]

There is much continuity between the 1910s and 1920s and the 1930s and 1940s with respect to the location of sports medicine practice. First aid was still given on the pitch or track, by volunteers and paid club doctors or school medical officers. Increasingly, however, this provision became formalised. Although practitioners were still often voluntary, the system that provided them was increasingly official. At the elite level, the medical provision at the Olympics increases, not only in terms of the facilities on offer in the host country (in this period usually including a dedicated hospital), but also in the numbers of staff brought with visiting teams. In professional sport, the attendance of a medical officer at matches or games gradually became compulsory.[23]

In (professional) Association Football the formalisation of medical services had been ongoing since at least 1912, when a court case ruled that professional footballers were manual labourers and should be covered under the 1911 National Insurance Act. This ruling meant that they were eligible for medical care and services part-sponsored by their employer (i.e. the

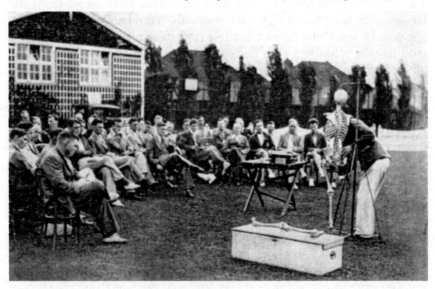

**3.** A lesson in 'Anatomy'. This photograph shows students at Loughborough College attending a lecture on 'Anatomy' in the late 1930s. This course was intended for men who wanted to become physical educationalists and physical trainers, and was organised by FAM Webster (1886–1949) – it was the first such course organised in Britain. It is likely that this photograph was taken by Webster himself (*c.* 1937, although it has proved impossible specifically to attribute it to him or any of the photographers he used).

club). As a consequence professional footballers were covered by legislation which did not apply to the amateur sportsperson.[24] At the same time, it is clear that football clubs invested in medical care above and beyond anything demanded by National Insurance regulations. For example, by the mid-1940s Southampton Football Club – then only a second division team – had an extensive medical advisory team (an orthopaedic surgeon, a general practitioner and a member of the Chartered Society of Physiotherapy). Their club treatment room was:

> equipped up to the standard of any hospital physical medicine department, possessing short-wave diathermy apparatus, radiant heat baths, infra-red lamps, thermostatically controlled wax baths, galvanic, faradic and sinusoidal tables, ultra-violet generators suitable for mass-irradiation, sling-and-pulley exercise apparatus, graduated weights suitable for muscle-resistance exercises, massage plinths, and surgical trolleys.[25]

This sort of provision was not exceptional; First Division Arsenal had by 1950 a Club Doctor and a 'fully equipped physiotherapy and rehabilitation department' including 'all the necessary apparatus for electrical treatment and remedial exercises'.[26] Serious treatment at the professional clubs still tended to be undertaken in general hospitals, but rehabilitation and training was, by the 1940s, almost entirely under the remit of the nominated (and usually voluntary) club doctor.[27] Certainly, by the 1940s, provision of medical care at professional football clubs easily surpassed the care one would expect for similar skilled manual labourers; for example at a small factory an employer of up to 500 people would be expected only to have a part-time doctor and ensure that there was a casualty room on-site for emergency injury treatment.[28] There was absolutely no question of employer-provided physiologists, UV light or heat baths for most manual workers in the 1940s or 1950s.

As the previous chapter discussed, much sports medicine practice is invisible to the historian, being part and parcel of everyday medical treatment, and not preserved in archives or readily available materials. Medical textbooks and articles, on the other hand, tend to represent an idealised version of medical provision. That said, what is clear is the emphasis on 'scientific training' which appears fundamental in theory, even if it was less consistently applied in practice. Virtually every textbook on sport or exercise physiology, and every training manual published in Britain took time to decry the 'backwards' or 'superstitious' or 'faddy' habits of other trainers:

> [s]ome of the old-time prejudices are still extant, and to them we have added some new fads and fancies of our own. The trouble is that new scientific principles, even when their value is fully proved do not easily overcome

custom. They may appeal to a man's logic and yet not conquer his deep-rooted convictions.[29]

This criticism, by the athlete and Olympic coach FAM Webster (1886–1949) is directed at the diet of athletes. He claims that two of the main reasons for such 'faddism' are that there is inadequate research, and that these fads use pseudo-scientific arguments (rather than appeals to tradition) in their adverts.[30] This general feeling of a need for more scientific research, alongside greater medical control and authority, is repeated in many texts.

The practice of sports medicine in sites away from the track and field was being forced by national events and concerns. Governmental intervention in sports had a direct influence, through the activities of school Medical Officers, on some medical care and screening for schoolchildren, as well as generally raising interest at local governmental and city council level into the provision of playing fields, subsidised gyms, and attendant services.[31] But it was governmental involvement in science and in medicine directly, as much as with sport, which broadened out the site of sports medicine in the 1930s and 1940s. More clinical medical laboratories were constructed, and closer affiliations created between universities and medical institutions.[32] Many of these new clinics and laboratories began to investigate questions of physiology. At the same time, the Medical Research Council (hence MRC) – originally formed to investigate tuberculosis – was reinvented as a central clearing house for tax-funded medical research providing new opportunities for research and experiment.[33]

As a consequence two new sites for sports medicine opened up. First was the laboratory. Although sports science and exercise physiology had been practised to a limited extent in British (and more in European) research institutes, the 1930s and 1940s saw a boom in studies of human muscle, cardiology, respiration, and so on. Secondly, sports medicine was increasingly being practised in the hospital – not as the inevitable treatment of sprains, strains and fractures, but as a specific (and later specialised) activity. The first sports clinics, often taking place at odd hours through the voluntary service of interested practitioners, began to appear in the 1940s.[34] Sport could also be a cure as well as a cause of ill-health; while the National Fitness Council and suchlike promoted generic ideas of health and fitness, in some sites across the UK sport was being used as a form of rehabilitation for wounded veterans. As a consequence, the 1940s saw the emergence of disability sport, a new, and sometimes challenging, version of the 'athletic body' (see below).

Along with the multiplying sites for sports medicine came an increase in the number and range of sports medicine practitioners. Despite the emerging structure of sports medicine a great deal remained voluntary; enthusiasts still offered their time as club doctors, or ran informal clinics for injured amateur sportsmen on Monday mornings.[35] But funding and new sites for practice also led to new practitioners. From the clinical side there were those whose specialisms, originally focused on soldiers, were a natural fit for sports medicine. Secondly there were the exercise physiologists and sports scientists, often established in university facilities. Some of these practitioners could reasonably be considered experts in sports medicine, and their number was added to as clubs sought doctors of their own, and as the medical teams attending the Olympics, or the Commonwealth Games (from 1930), expanded. Likewise, auxiliary medical staff increased; physiotherapists, masseurs, even nutritionists began to appear in lists of support staff for various sports teams.

The previous chapter looked for organising themes in a period without institutions, or organisations. This chapter is interested instead in seeking out the sources of authority immediately before the foundation of the first British sports medicine organisation. In an earlier period such authority was largely vested in theories – theories of sport, of physiology, of bodily function, and ethics – which could be used as rough and ready tools to establish orthodoxy in sports medicine practice. While moderation and individuality were still strong rhetorical tools in the 1930s and 1940s, authority itself began to be invested elsewhere than in theory; increasingly it lay in organisations, individuals, and 'institutions' (both real and metaphorical). This is a time period of fewer consensuses than the period 1900–27, with regular debates in the medical, scientific, sporting, and public arenas about various aspects of sports medicine, from the measurement of fitness to the Athlete's Heart to the use of monkey gland extracts by professional footballers. These debates are characteristic of, and evidence for, the changing identity of the athlete, as well as the emergence of a specialism – a struggle for authority within and between sporting and medical groups which gradually resolved itself through the formation of 'official' organisations.

### The Olympics and international sports medicine

A great deal of British sports medicine practice, particularly in the very late 1920s and 1930s, was influenced by international developments. The increased interest in national fitness was certainly not confined to inter-war Britain, as across Europe governments considered the role of physical activity and sports in creating a strong nation. Between 1937 and 1938 the League of Nations conducted meetings and conferences and produced policy documents relating to physical education and fitness, a process involving several British doctors and scientists, including some from the MRC.[36] The outcomes of these meetings were cautious – exercise should only be undertaken under medical supervision, '[n]o one should engage in strenuous training and competitive exercises without a medical examination', and '[s]trenuous exercise should be avoided during menstruation' (*pace* later research in Britain).[37] That there is a division by this point between sport for general fitness, and elite sport is made explicit, as the League insists that '[t]he aim of physical education should be not to develop 'champions' but to benefit the whole community'.[38]

Biomedical events at the Olympic Games also influenced British sports medicine, as they usually involved British scientists and doctors as well as the bodies of British athletes, and much of this research was inspired by FIMS. The consolidation of sports medicine as a distinct medical specialty, at the international (mostly European) scale was indicated by the formation of FIMS in 1928. The seeds of FIMS were sown at an association of physicians for the promotion of athletic exercises (*Deutscher Ärztebund zur Förderung der Leibesübungen* f.1924) in Germany.[39] This German 'early start' in sports medicine has been highlighted by other historians and will be briefly discussed below, but it was Switzerland who probably had the first sports medicine organisation (a '"Sports-medical Committee" was formed within the Swiss Association of physical education') and it was a Swiss doctor, Professor W Knoll, who chaired the first meeting of FIMS.[40] In coincidence with the 1928 Winter Olympics in St Moritz, 33 (or 50 in some reports) doctors representing nearly a dozen countries discussed sports medicine and agreed the aims and objectives of the *Association Internationale Médico-Sportive* (AIMS) which became FIMS in 1934.[41]

There were no British doctors on the original committee presided over by Knoll. But one of the key participants, the Dutch Professor of Physiology Frederik Jacobus Johannes Buytendijk (1887–1974), trained under AV Hill in the 1910s.[42] As a member of the new FIMS executive committee Buytendijk was nominated to organise the First International Congress on Sports Medicine, which was planned to be held at the same time as the summer Olympics in Amsterdam in 1932. Nearly 300 people from 20 nations attended the Congress, and Buytendijk was subsequently elected as president of FIMS.[43] The organisation's initial aims were three-fold: to promote scientific research; to promote the study of physical education (in co-operation with sports organisations); and to organise conferences and congresses.

The activity of FIMS was disrupted by World War II and, despite the ambition of some members, the early period (to the late 1940s) was very much one of co-ordination and consolidation. It was not until 1952 that the IOC 'recognised the FIMS as the designated competent international organisation for biological and medical research related to medicine and sport and the medical care of the athlete'.[44] (This was the same year that Porritt and Abrahams formed Britain's first sports medicine organisation, which itself started life firmly associated with – indeed with the same postal address as – the British Olympic Association). Yet, even before its official recognition by the IOC, FIMS played an important role in the development of sports medicine in Britain. Its semi-regular congresses, and their varied key topics provided space for the few enthusiasts globally (though mostly in Europe and North America) to meet, discuss, and collaborate. In its first year FIMS was also instrumental in the introduction of a novel and extensive set of biomedical tests and experiments conducted on Olympic athletes (and more on this below).

As the 1928 *BMJ* editorial quoted at the beginning of this chapter makes clear, it was Germany who was considered Britain's main 'competitor' in terms of developments in sports medicine and exercise physiology. It is, of course, debatable how much Germany's 'lead' was measured in research and clinical practice, and how much of it was post-World War I sensitivity to Teutonic advancement.[45] The two seminal histories of German sports medicine by Hoberman and Heiss present us with an impressive list of 'firsts' or achievements:

1904, first use of term 'sports physician',

1912, first official sports physician conference held in Oberhof/ Thüringen,

1919, first University lecture course on sports medicine – 'The Hygiene of Sports and Performance',

1920, first sports college with a sports medicine curriculum.[46]

There is certainly much in this list which could be used to incite anxiety or jealousy in 'enemy' nations, or by historians to make the case for Germany as the premier sports medicine nation.

Yet it is revealing to look at the similarities between Germany and Britain; in both nations there was strong resistance *from within the medical profession* against recognising sports medicine as a medical specialty (resistance which continued in Britain until the end of the century). Heiss categorises German sports medicine as being made up of three distinct periods: 1912–25, application of general medical theories to athletes; 1925–55, gradual increase in interest and research in the specifics of the athletic body and exercise physiology; *c.* 1965, the appearance of sports medicine as a distinct specialism.[47] The previous chapter (*c.* 1900–27) told of Britain's sports medicine when it was the application of general medical theories to athletes. This chapter (1928–52) discusses the increase in research and understanding specifically relating to athletics and athletes' bodies. Therefore, this development is roughly in line with Heiss's chronology. Once again, it is important to acknowledge that a lack of institutions or organisations does not always indicate a lack of practice or interest – massage proved that point in Chapter 2. Undoubtedly Germany gained institutions, academics and organisational outlets for sports medicine years, in some cases decades, before the UK. It is also true that German scholars produced some pioneering work in sports medicine and exercise physiology. But, when grossly periodised, British sports medicine as a research practice and as a concept kept rough pace with Germany; it was the 1930s and 1940s where concerted efforts began to be made in Britain to research the athlete and his injuries specifically, rather than apply 'general' biomedical knowledge to his training and treatment.

Of course, Germany was not representative of the rest of the world. The USA's institutions and organisations came even later, despite that nation's evolving sporting precedence. Nonetheless, it was the second US-based Olympic Games, in Los Angeles in 1932, which pioneered the use of an Olympic Village – giving new structure and impetus to medical provision at the Games. At the previous Olympic Games in Amsterdam (1928) the pattern of medical provision was much like those seen in Chapter 2. Services were co-ordinated between the local Municipal Medical Service and the Red Cross. All work, even that of the employees of the Municipal Medical Service was voluntary, bar expenses.[48] 'Extensive measures were taken' for the marathon, run at around 3pm and the total medical staff was numbered in the dozens.[49] Most significant, though, were the physiological studies organised by Buytendijk, which will be discussed below.

Four years later, the Organising Committee for the 1932 Los Angeles Games deliberately set out to create the most 'detailed medical organisation for the care of sick or injured athletes'.[50] Support was provided, as always, by the local medical service and the Red Cross – but also from private physicians and surgeons. This work was co-ordinated by an unprecedented 15 advisory committees: Medical; Surgical; Eye, ear, nose and throat; Dental; Women's; Research; Lung; Heart; Dermatology; Psychiatry; X-ray; Nursing; Physiotherapy; Equipment; and Hospitalisation. Although at previous Olympic Games the central focus for provision had been the main stadium itself, now it shifted to the residential village, where a Village Hospital was built. Novel too was the Medical Committee's interest in aspects of public health and environmental engineering, with a Sanitary Inspector at the village. In particular, athlete's foot was considered as a health risk, and the local County Health Officer and County Chemist conducted trials of fungicidal treatment.[51]

The marathon commanded greatest supervision, as had become traditional, and the entrants were examined by 'four heart specialists in addition to the chief surgeon and his assistants', an examination which included urinary analyses, and heart, lung and blood pressure tests.[52] To give a perspective on the vast medical staffing: as well as a Medical Director and Assistant Medical Director, there was a Chief Medical Consultant, and a 'Medical Advisory Board' of sixteen MDs (all male), eighteen honorary surgeons, and hundreds of further advisers, including twenty-one volunteer dentists, and 'foreign consultants' from entrant countries, including Britain.[53] The total number of athletes treated in the hospital was 574, including fifty-six women.

Berlin was not to be outdone in 1936. Once more, local medical services and the Red Cross co-operated to staff eleven first-aid rooms, a two-storey stadium hospital with twenty-seven rooms and further emergency rooms and medical depots.[54] One hundred and seventy-one physicians were supported by at least 200 volunteer first-aiders. The Berlin Olympic Committee's report makes much of their very 'modern' telephone network connecting all these services; for face-to-face communication, they also introduced a medical translation service in order to 'devel[op] closer connections with the foreign doctors, and of enabling their wishes regarding conferences and tours through scientific institutions to be granted'.[55] However close and friendly the relationships between the medical staff accompanying the Olympic teams became, many were shattered during the conflict that followed.

When the next Olympic Games took place in London, in 1948, the pattern of local medical and voluntary first-aid provision was preserved, although military services also played a very significant role, as well as heavy involvement from private firms, such as Boots Ltd.[56] In part this was a consequence of the extreme financial restrictions on the Games, colloquially known as the 'austerity games'. The Medical Committee for the London Olympics was formed in the Autumn of 1946, and consisted of many names later to become key players in British sports medicine: Abrahams, Porritt, and Brigadier Glyn Hughes. A V Hill was invited onto the committee as was Dr Louise Albertine Winner, the latter specifically asked because the executive board thought that there ought to be a woman on the Committee.[57]

Despite the organisational and fiscal restrictions (the Medical Committee were given a budget of around £1000 to cover the medical costs of over 4000 athletes and other team members) the Medical Services at the 1948 games were at least comparable to previous and subsequent Games. First aid was available at all sites, and physiotherapy and minor medical treatment at all major competition and residential areas; the Football Association were approached to provide suitably trained physiotherapists, and some sports – notably boxing – also provided trained and experienced medical personnel for their events. The Committee spent £15 on case cards for the reporting of injuries, around 550 of which were returned, mostly reporting minor injuries such as cuts and abrasions, as well as 25 cases of gastroenteritis. The Committee noted that '[i]t is of interest ... that in a country with a climate such as England's both sunburn and insect bites produced a noticeable number of patients [3 and 21]'.[58]

Although money was tight the Committee attempted to provide as modern a service as possible. In February 1947 they wrote to Sir Alexander Fleming to ask his opinion on whether penicillin should be given as a standard treatment (alongside or instead of anti-tetanus serum) to all injured athletes.[59] In the spring of 1948 they arranged for beds to be put aside for possible psychiatric patients, in particular boxers suffering from the much-debated punch-drunk syndrome.[60] While these may seem commonplace arrangements for a modern Olympics, they are both evidence of a connection to the latest research in physiology and medicine – as is the appointment of AV Hill, a man, after all, without a medical qualification, not a member of a sports organisation, and with no experience of mass medical provision at a sporting event. Hill's appointment can only have been on the strength of his expertise in the special physiology of the athletic body, and as such reflects the gradual shift from normality to supernormality which is traced in this chapter.

By the time organisational normality had returned to the Games at the 1952 Helsinki Olympics, the growth patterns of the inter-war Games were solidified. The Helsinki Organising Committee set up a Medical Committee in 1951, and had an extensive staff of medical specialists and advisers on a variety of Executive and Advisory Boards well in advance of the Opening Ceremony. The Helsinki Committee laid emphasis on auxiliary treatment – Head Nurses were in charge of procuring supplies, while physiotherapy and remedial services were central to the overall provision of medical services. Specialist training was provided to the medical staff:

> Although a large proportion of the medical personnel engaged for the Games were former athletes or in other ways well acquainted with sports, informative and educational occasions were arranged shortly before the Games, separately for medical officers and nurses. The subjects dealt with were the general organisation of the Games, the main features of the medical services, the compulsory medical examinations, the treatment of sportsmen's injuries, and sportsmen's sicknesses from the physician's point of view.[61]

The Medical Committee also set down minimum standards for the services they intended to supply, e.g. one first-aid room at every venue, artificial respiration systems at all water sports venues, and so on.[62] Four hundred and nineteen medical staff were hired – although this includes all auxiliaries and administrative personnel – treating 1136 athletes (and a total of 3244 people including officials and spectators).[63]

The effect on British sports medicine of this increase in medical provision and organisation internationally can really only be a matter of speculation. British athletes will certainly have experienced this increasing medical intervention and coverage. Even if they never became sick or injured, the imposition of measures such as anti-athlete's foot treatment (including footbaths) would be noticeable, although the 'compulsory' treatment was often avoidable.[64] So, too, the meetings, workshops and conferences (with medical consultants and translators) organised around the Olympiads by FIMS and similar organisations, facilitated communication.

But alongside the co-ordination, communication and regularisation of services, came a second trend in Olympic sports medicine, which was of great significance to the practice and structure of British sports medicine, and that was research. Starting in the comprehensive physiological research organised by Buytendijk in 1928, the Olympics became the site of direct investigation of the athletic body.[65] Initially this was limited to the literal site of the Games themselves; eventually it would expand so that the IOC itself became a gatekeeper, arbitrator and financier of research chronologically and geographically distanced from the immediate practice of the Olympic Games themselves. Strangely, the 1932 Los Angeles Olympic Games bucked this trend – despite having a research sub-committee, the Executive Medical Advisory Committee concluded that:

> in view of the splendid work which had already been done for thousands of athletes, and on account of the short space of time during which research work could be carried on, the varied nationalities represented, the opposition on the part of some athletes, and the difficulties of obtaining proper facilities and apparatus convenient to the athletic contests, it would be unwise to attempt medical research at this time.[66]

Several organisational factors made research problematic in 1948, but in 1928, 1936 and 1952 physiological or epidemiological research on athletes was a prominent part of the Olympic medical programme.

Non-treatment medical interventions had already taken place – for example the screening for marathon and cycling – but the research in 1928 and afterwards was different. This was no longer protective and preventive screening, but active medical research, not to preserve the health of the individual participants, but to create general knowledge about exercise physiology and the athlete's body, *distinct from the non-athletes' body*. And this research had a direct impact on sports medicine in Britain, as British researchers took part, including AV Hill and two physiologists from

Manchester, Professor Bramwell and Dr Ellis who travelled to Amsterdam to undertake cardiological and blood pressure research.[67]

## Constructing the 'athletic body'

Research was also being undertaken within the UK. In 1928 Adolphe Abrahams conducted a thorough examination of 'all the leading athletes in the country who were probable and possible candidates for Olympic representation at Amsterdam' which included 'psychical . . . physical and anatomical details'.[68] Abrahams' conclusion was that psychological factors played a determining role in sporting success, because:

> when one reached the very cream of athletic prowess there was nothing by which to distinguish the heart, the lungs, the muscular development of the superman from those of any well-developed youth leading a healthy life and taking a fair amount of exercise.[69]

Abrahams' work illustrates precisely the shift from normal to supernormal over the period considered in this chapter, when he refers to the 'very cream' of British athletes in 1928 as 'only well-developed youth', but by 1951 he is writing instead of the 'constitutional hypertrophy of the super athlete'.[70]

This emerging divide between the 'normal' and the 'athlete' was not entirely desirable – Abrahams regularly stated that he thought they ought to be one and the same thing. Nonetheless, it was increasingly recognised, even by those who disapproved like Abrahams, that the athlete was something new, something different. In later years Abrahams' letters were a regular feature in the columns of national newspapers defending the Olympic failures of British athletes, on the grounds that the Olympic elite were at a 'preposterous standard', and that British teams were doing as well as could be expected, given that they were essentially 'well-developed youths' and not 'super-athletes'.[71]

Bramwell and Ellis were also interested in constitutional hypertrophy; their study of Olympic athletes in 1928 was much larger than Abrahams', involving 202 runners. The puzzle that particularly fascinated them was the question 'what . . . constitute[s] a successful Marathon runner?'; was it, they speculated, 'something in the liver, or possibly a psychological factor' which enabled him to run such a distance?[72] Was his stable pulse rate evidence of particularly strong emotional continence? Perhaps unintentionally, Bramwell and Ellis identify the runner as *different*. Their tone of voice suggests he is super- rather than ab-normal, but he is different not only from the lay public, but even from other athletes.[73] Research at the Olympic Games was therefore valuable not because it provided access to a large number of guinea pigs for physiological experiments, but because it gave access to a specific breed of guinea pigs, i.e. elite sporting bodies – bodies which were increasingly being categorised by doctors and scientists as a discrete sort of clinical entity, a distinctive and unique human *type*.

In discussing research and exercise physiology we come to a thematic and semantic difficulty, and that is the distinction between sports medicine and sports science. Whatever the developments in sports science and exercise physiology as theory and knowledge, these still had to be interpreted to become sports medicine practice, and it is this process of mediation and practice which is the core interest of this book. The period between 1928 and 1952 saw an increase in the organisations, institutions and individuals involved in this mediation; from the lone enthusiasts of the early century to sub-committees and devolved branches of larger organisations – e.g. the MRC – through to a specific, independent, sports medicine organisation. As a consequence, there were at minimum dozens, and more realistically, hundreds, of individual scientists, doctors, sportsmen, civil servants and the like, engaged in this process of interpretation and application.

Just two men, however, dominate and best *characterise* sports medicine and sports science in the first half of the twentieth century, and they are Adolphe Abrahams and AV Hill, whose biographies are outlined in Boxes 2 and 4.[74] Abrahams is without doubt a Sports *Doctor*, involved in practical application as well as research, and his work will continue to be discussed below, and in subsequent chapters. Hill, on the other hand, despite his personal interest in athletes, is the epitome of a Sports *Scientist*. As the amount of research into sporting performance and the athletic body increased in this period, so did the number of organisations involved in mediating and interpreting any findings, and since the output of the former certainly affected the work of the latter it is worth sketching some of the key research.

Hill's Nobel Prize-winning research was into the function of muscles, and from the 1920s he published on aerobic and anaerobic exercise, the role of oxygen and lactic acid in muscle function, and outlined the concept of 'oxygen debt'. Important too was Hill's work defining systems of measurement – for example the concept of $VO_2$max, which is still used in athletic assessment and experiments.[75] Hill also acted to popularise, or at least make reputable, the study of exercise and athletes.[76] Hill's work took place against a background of expansion in physiology and its division into sub-disciplines. Research into basic human physiology provided information of use to athletes, including continued attention to the physiology of muscles and nerves, and the function of the pulmonary and cardiological system (including the perennial problem of the Athlete's Heart).[77] The 1930s and 1940s also saw a great deal of output on the chemistry of life – including the ongoing 'discovery' and synthesis of vitamins and their role in human diets, as well as the identification, extraction and even simulation of human hormones.[78] Even the most 'advanced' or cutting-edge of this research could still be used in practice; as Abrahams wrote in 1928, the question which interested the athlete was '[c]an the physiologist discover something which will enable him to knock off a vital fifth of a second from his time on the track?'.[79]

One particularly scandalous example of the absorption of 'fashionable' physiological findings was the Monkey Gland controversy of the late 1930s. Although (or perhaps because) the story was particularly tabloid-friendly it is difficult to exactly establish what happened. Hormonal extracts had been used by athletes worldwide since at least the late nine-teenth century.[80] Likewise gland extracts to 'vitalise' (and usually sexually invigorate) middle-aged men had been licitly or illicitly taken in Britain for years.[81] In the late 1930s Frank Buckley, the manager of the (First Division) Wolverhampton Wanderers Football Club, allegedly arranged for the club doctor to inject the players with monkey-gland extracts. While it was possible at that time to get hold of, for example, solutions of testo-sterone or other hormones, there is little evidence that Buckley actually did dope his players. Some subsequent reports have claimed that this was nothing more than a flu inoculation and some morale-boosting PR. Nonetheless, the gland stories continued to run, Buckley's wife apparently telling the press that it had improved his bedroom technique, and team captain Billy Wright writing that he slipped his 'capsule' of gland treat-ment to his 'family feline' which became 'the prize cat of the area!'.[82]

The use of glands and hormones was discussed in other sports, and apparently several football (and cricket) clubs took up the practice.[83] Eventually a question was asked in Parliament about the heath risks of a 'gland final' in Association Football, and the British Medical Association resolved to investigate the matter.[84] World War II intervened and the investigation never took place; by the time doping in sports was a serious issue again, in the 1950s, the context in which rules and regulations were needed was quite different (see the next chapter). The 'gland expert' engaged by Buckley, Mr A Menzies Sharp, argued in the 1930s that hor-mones were no different to any other form of legal enhancement (a senti-ment shared by many of the present generation of sports sociologists):

> It should be remembered that the treatment is given several days before, not just prior to, the event. Gland treatment is not a method of doping; it is as much a part of training as exercises or ray treatment. [85]

So Menzies Sharp was working in the transitional period between the normal athlete and the athlete as super-, sub- or ab-normal; later the chemical purity of the sportsman had to be maintained to reinforce a new clinical object – the athletic body.[86]

The emergence of the athlete as a distinct patient type is evident in other areas of sports medicine, including everything from the latest cardiological findings to basic treatments for muscular strains and sprains. The Athlete's Heart re-emerges as a clinical phenomenon; by 1928 there was general consensus among physiologists, doctors and sportsmen alike that exercise could not harm the normal heart. Athlete's hearts might hypertrophy in proportion with their muscular development, but dilatation and 'strain' were characteristic only of hearts with a congenital weakness or predisposition to disease. By the 1950s the *disproportionately* enlarged athlete's heart had become an advantage for the athlete.[87] So between 1928 and 1952 the 'Athlete's Heart' became a clinical entity for a second time; while it had been feared as pathology by the Victorians and then dismissed as a myth by the Edwardians, by the mid-century it was recognised as a physiological adaptation – evidence of supernormal rather than abnormal status. While the heart still retains its iconic status, other body systems began to be drawn into debates with similar trajectories.[88] There was also an increase in the articles published on injuries and diseases with specific athletic aetiology.[89]

The fundamental dilemma here, as I argue is always the case for sports medicine, is the division between normal and abnormal – not just in symptoms and clinical presentation but also in activity and environment. If running the marathon is to be considered a 'normal' human activity, then the anatomical or physiological changes induced must also be considered as part of a 'normal' range of human reactions. Alternatively, if marathon running is to be considered an exceptional or abnormal activity, then the physiological consequences of running ought not be judged against the clinical indicators of 'normal' behaviour. Instead the marathon is a special activity producing bodily conditions that are both *special* but also *contextually normal*; there is not one normal physiology, there are many. This latter approach, of course, highlights the athletic body as 'special', as distinct from mainstream medicine as the medical 'body' of the child, or the elderly person, or the pregnant woman.

### Inventing sports medicine

While the leading lights of British sports medicine continued to resist the notion that sports medicine should be a recognised medical specialty until well into the 1980s and 1990s they still contributed to a medical (and lay) understanding of the athletic body as special and requiring special consideration by specialists. This shift is gradual between 1928 and 1952; when

Heald's seminal *Injuries in Sport* was published in 1931, the *Lancet* review, while positive, also points out that many of these injuries can occur away from the track, field or ring:

> The title of this book is unfair to its scope. Bodily injuries are not, in this country at least, primarily associated with sport, and it may be doubted whether the injuries sustained as a result of sports differ in any essential way from other injuries.[90]

But Heald's was just the first in an increasing number of similar publications. While Heald did make use of the pioneering exercise physiology of Hill, these early publications followed on from Romer's work (see above) in their concentration on the primary application of biomedical knowledge to the direct and immediate treatment and prevention of injuries.

Issues of enhancement and policing were not ignored, however; war once again sharpened the government and public's focus on the 'fitness' (or otherwise) of the nation, and in the 1930s and 1940s ideas of physical fitness, exercise and sport became tightly conflated. Even in this positive atmosphere some voices of caution were raised, for example Dr Heald, the 'inventor' of the idea of sports injuries in Britain, gave an extremely ambiguous account of the value of sport in a 1934 lecture and article on 'Physical Exercise and Sport as Preventatives of Disease'.[91] This tension between exercise and fitness on the one hand, and notions of stress, strain, overwork and sports injury on the other, is particularly important when state intervention is in question; to what degree should a government promote the rewards of sport, to what degree offset the risks? This is an issue which became most pressing after the founding of the NHS, and in particular with the leisure boom at the end of the century, discussed in Chapter 5.

In the last chapter we saw how medical professionals claimed authority over the body 'at risk' of sports injury – i.e. the school child or the person with a hidden disease. In the 1980s and 1990s this authority was successfully expanded to the whole population using similar arguments about risk and reward, but in the 1940s, without an obviously self-defining group of experts to claim that role, the plea remained more generic – for 'more research' rather than 'more authority'. Heald added that:

> If the modern enthusiasm for physical training is to be developed on sound lines it must be based on a much more accurate knowledge of human physiology than is at present available, especially of the functions of the liver and the lymphatic and sympathetic systems.[92]

Such a plea for more research, more specialist information, is a common theme in this period.

So this interest, regardless of whether it was based on positive expectations (for example, increasing the fitness of the nation) or fears (for example, about sickness and injury), led to increasing interest in, and funding for, exercise science and sports medicine. It also saw new clinical and laboratory attention paid to the peculiarities and needs of all sports.[93] While the marathon was still central, articles (and books) were published on the injuries of cricket, the athlete's knee, tennis elbow, and a host of other conditions and activities.[94]

Nor was this medical attention entirely created within the laboratory or clinic; increasingly sportsmen and sports organisations solicited medical advice and supervision.[95] The most obvious example of this is the case of boxing. A more detailed account of the medicalisation of boxing is given elsewhere.[96] In brief: two factors coalesced to put pressure on the British Boxing Board of Control (hence: BBBC, f.1929) regarding the introduction of medical controls. A series of significant articles were published in this period on the medical and neurological sequelae of boxing, and the experience of war had increased research on traumatic, combative head injuries.[97] The BBBC appointed a Chief Medical Officer in 1946, and four years later introduced a comprehensive system of medical supervision, inspection and record cards.[98] Medical supervision had already been present for amateur boxing, as evidenced by the Olympics of 1948 where the Medical Committee actually relied on the Amateur Boxing Association to provide qualified medical supervision for all the Olympic bouts.

The BBBC ramped up its medical activities in the 1950s; the nature of boxing makes it a sport which continues to be controversial. We can speculate that the relatively 'early' uptake of formalised medical supervision may have been a defensive reaction – creating an expert body in-house, before any such body could emerge from without. Other, more conventional possibilities are simply public or medical pressure on boxing, which is viewed as a particularly dangerous or violent sport, and/or the economic aspect – as a commercial enterprise boxing could afford doctors, while many other sports could not.

Before considering further the growth of organisations, institutions and other 'mediators' of sports science and sports medicine, it is worth acknowledging a new relationship between sport and medicine, and that is the growth of sport as a curative and rehabilitative treatment. Doctors had previously prescribed a brisk walk, sea-bathing or mountain air to various categories of patient, and, as the last chapter showed, massage and movement had become mainstream treatment. In the 1940s though, an entirely new strand of sports-as-therapy appeared. Just as work on Athlete's Heart was provoked by wartime desires and funding, so this novel avenue was also a consequence of the desire for rehabilitation for thousands of disabled servicemen. Much of this development took place at the Spinal Injury Centre at the Stoke Mandeville Hospital in Aylesbury. The work done there was revolutionary, and it introduced an entirely new (to Britain) form of sport, later to become the Paralympics.[99]

When the centre opened in 1944, the traditional form of 'activity' therapy for people who were physically disabled was work therapy, often manual work such as sewing or pottery. Such activity had a two-fold purpose, firstly to aid physical and mental rehabilitation, and secondly to act as retraining, allowing the disabled veteran to re-enter society as an economically productive citizen. The Director (Sir) Ludwig Guttman (1899–1980) introduced a new scheme of rehabilitation, where 'clinical sport' played a role as remedial treatment – to 'mobilise dormant neuromuscular mechanisms in the normal part of the body to compensate for the lost function in the paralyzed part'.[100] Importantly, this sport was often to be competitive, on the grounds that this challenge encouraged men to do their best, and had a profound psychological effect, 'prevent[ing] the paralyzed from resigning themselves to their disability'.[101] This was not the first use of sport as a moral and psychological curative, or a means of reintegration for marginalised groups but it is significant for its overwhelmingly medical discourse and government funding.[102] Significant too was the formalization of the sporting competition as the Stoke Mandeville Games in 1948. At the chronological close of this chapter, 1952, the Stoke Mandeville Games opened to international competition when a group of 'paralyzed Dutch ex-servicemen' arrived to take part. International participation increased, and the Games were rechristened as the Paralympics in 1985.[103]

Disability sport poses obvious questions about (ab)normality; as the Games enlarged, new, complicated categories of sportsman/woman were introduced, as physical, sensory and mental disabilities were ranked and categorised, ostensibly to ensure fair play. Comparatively, able-bodied sport, with its distinctions only of gender, age, weight, and experience is more straightforward. A full examination of disabled sports medicine is outwith the remit of this book, but one common theme between able-bodied and disabled sport can be drawn out; disabled sportsmen started as 'battling soldiers' using sport as a therapy for social reintegration and physical healing. Through the mid-century, they became sportsmen and women in their own right – disabled athletes and then disabled professionals.[104] That their 'special' bodies required 'special' rules, supervision, and treatment reflects in part the experiences of able-bodied sportsmen and women, where the athlete emerged as a discrete physical type.

One further difference between Guttman's work and earlier examples of disability sport or sport-as-therapy is that while the latter were usually philanthropically organised, the rehabilitation at the Stoke Mandeville Centre was largely state-funded. Changes in government funding for scientific and medical work had a significant impact on the development of sports medicine as a body of knowledge, and a discipline, not least the straightforward economic boost to physiological research in the UK. These changes went hand-in-hand with broader cultural and political pressures of war. As has been shown extensively for the Boer War, military conflict provokes questions and fears about the physical fitness of a nation – not just its soldiers but also the resilience and health of its civilian population.[105] A renewed interest, then, in physical fitness, exercise, and health fed through into the practice of sports medicine. Even the experience of rationing played a role in constructing knowledge about athletes' bodies, requiring, as it did, further research on diet, nutrition, metabolism and caloric requirements.[106]

A great deal of this funding came through the Medical Research Council, which was founded in 1913 as the Medical Research *Committee*, using funds secured from provisions in the 1911 National Health Insurance Act. Early plans for research, which included a department of Applied Physiology, were dropped with the start of World War I. The Committee was 'relaunched' as a Council in 1920, with a relationship to the Department of Science and Industrial Research and the Ministry of Health (founded in 1915 and 1919 respectively). Its remit was to ensure 'proper' scientific independence from government.[107]

Physiology and applied physiology appear and disappear as core parts of the MRC's work. The Department of Applied Physiology existed between 1914 and 1928, then a Department of Physiology between 1930 and 1931.[108] In 1945 two physiology departments, 'Physiology and Pharmacy' and 'Applied Physiology' were in place, although the latter was dropped in 1948 and replaced in 1950 by a dedicated Division of Human Physiology.[109] This Division played a vital role in the investigation of athletic performance at altitude, a key issue in the next chapter, but up until 1952 there was only a limited amount of research directly into sport or athletics by the MRC. Generally, sports medicine-relevant work consisted either of research into fitness or what we can term 'basic' physiological research.

Between 1928 and 1952, the MRC organised or funded research into the sports medicine-relevant areas of: steroids; the metabolism of carbohydrates; the synthesis and utility of vitamins; respiratory and cardio-pulmonary research; the role of sex hormones; exercise and fatigue (though this was mostly related to industry); and 'environmental physiology' (i.e. human reactions to heat, cold, etc.). Although the MRC was supposed to ensure distance between scientific and medical research and the government, an increasing governmental interest in sport and physical exercise still influenced the MRC. The 1937 Physical Training and Recreation Act stated a desire to increase physical exercise and recreation facilities, so the Board of Education specifically asked the MRC to provide advice (and therefore do research) on the medical aspects of fitness.[110] A Physical Exercise Research Committee was formed, but had barely started work before World War II curtailed its activity.

The 1937 Act also inspired the CCPR to form a Medical Advisory Committee, although this was also short-lived, lasting only until 1939. Despite this, it managed to create two sub-committees, delineate a definition of 'fitness' as applied to the population, and conduct an investigation into the suitability of sport for women. (Abrahams acted as chair on the sub-committee on the effects of exercise on women.) The work of this latter committee largely consisted of a series of questionnaires and surveys sent to female athletes, women's sports clubs, and doctors, the great majority of which, apparently to the dismay of the committee, were returned fully supporting exercise (even violent exercise) for women.[111] In fact, by 1939, although 'the sub-committee had endeavoured to obtain adverse criticism on violent exercise for women and girls', it had done so 'without success'.[112]

The competitive aspects of sport, however, still posed a challenge to images of national womanhood, as one witness to the committee criticised 'certain first-class tennis players who entered tournament after tournament until they became aggressive and hysterical'.[113] While the medical witnesses appeared to be more conservative about female sport than sportswomen themselves, women still solicited the advice, support, and even control of doctors. For example, the 'president of the Southern Counties Amateur Swimming Club, Manageress of the women's team to the Empire Games in 1937/8, diving and swimming champion' made a case for the need for proper medical certification of 'fitness to participate' to prevent overstrain in female swimmers.[114]

The other sub-committee of the National Fitness Council was that on 'the criteria of fitness'.[115] 'Fitness' is an extraordinarily nebulous term throughout the twentieth century (see Chapter 6). Certainly, those involved in state-sponsored fitness schemes and committees held a very holistic definition of fitness, involving psychological and personality traits as well as physical characteristics, as an article in the *British Medical Journal* (1938) suggests:

The aim . . . of the present campaign for physical fitness is . . . to achieve a harmony of motion, a grace of carriage, a pride of body, a mental concentration and quickness of reactions, and a happiness and contentment which characterise the really fit.[116]

Other sources tended towards the more functional aspects of fitness, as a summary article in the *Annual Review of Physiology* (1946) makes clear:

> the fit man shows: lower oxygen consumption; slower pulse rate during wor!. ; lower systolic blood pressure during work; larger stroke volume; lower blood lactate during work; and faster return of blood pressure and pulse rate to resting value after work. If both are performing the same work which neither can sustain in a steady state, the fit man shows: longer duration of effort before exhaustion; higher oxygen consumptions; somewhat slower maximal pulse rate; larger stroke volume; higher blood lactate; and faster return of blood pressure to normal after work.[117]

Although the exact difference between the fit and the unfit, the abnormal and the super-normal, the athlete and the well-trained youth, may not be clear, the increased state interest in 'national fitness', research in exercise physiology, and raised world sporting standards meant that distinctions between the normal man and the athlete became more obvious.[118]

War-time contingencies certainly had a direct effect on the provision of services of use to the athlete and those with sports injuries. As Dr RS Woods (see previous chapter) wrote: 'under the Emergency Hospital Scheme, hospital facilities for physical medicine have multiplied many times'.[119] Some hospitals also organised 'Accident Services' which concentrated on orthopaedic treatment of 'certain types of cases previously dealt with in casualty', particularly fractures; in at least one instance, this rearrangement seems to have given impetus to the provision of an informal sports clinic within the newly formed NHS.[120] Although rest continued to be prescribed as treatment for sprains and strains, the trend, as discussed in the previous chapter, had shifted to physiotherapy and active exercise treatment:

> There has . . . been a wide break away from the traditional doctrine of long rest, a faulty outcome of the teaching that 'repair is but the repetition of growth' and 'rest is necessary antecedent to the healthy accomplishment of both repair and growth'.[121]

Some of this was facilitated by the introduction (by the Royal College of Surgeons and Royal College of Physicians) of a Diploma in Physical Medicine in 1945.[122]

Although often short-lived, the organisations, institutions, divisions and committees briefly discussed above, were part of a broader trend in the relationship between government/state and both sport and medicine.[123] Increasingly interventionist, the governmental process of supplying and organising funding also imposed systems of bureaucratic order and organisation. In the story of British sports medicine this creates two major influences – firstly, a 'habit' or culture of organisation, and, secondly, a much broader body of men (and rarely women) with a formal expertise in sport and medicine. Figure 3 shows young men at a CCPR-approved training course at Loughborough around 1938 learning to be Physical Training instructors; the lesson shown is in *Anatomy*, and the course handbooks clearly show how much physiology and medicine were included in this training.

### Conclusion: idealised citizens

So sports medicine was served and affected by new organisations, new institutions, new ideas and new funding – what effect did this have on the athlete and his body? There have been changes in provision, even for the amateur, Saturday-afternoon sportsman – aside from the increased access to health care provided by the NHS, he is somewhat more likely to be treated by a doctor, consultant or surgeon with an interest in sports medicine, or who has read specialist texts like *Injuries in Sport* (this level of expertise having only really been available to the elite or professional athlete in previous years). His treatment, informed by war, of exercise therapy, physiotherapy, orthopaedic surgery, rehabilitation, etc., will now more often reflect the most pioneering sort of sports medicine treatment available prior to World War I. The sport he engages in is also now part of a (sometimes) nationally important web of health and fitness. As well as the increasing awareness of the needs of sportsmen, and growing provision of open spaces for physical exercise, there is also a change in the athletic body at the end of this period – it is no longer 'merely' the fit and healthy 'normal' man. While the superstars of the late nineteenth and early twentieth century had attracted special attention, the rhetoric of sports medicine still figured the athlete as 'normal man' – and sporting wonders as abnormals and freaks (especially bodybuilders).

The change between 1928 and 1952 is incomplete, but is perhaps best proven by those who clung to the notion that the athlete *should* be normal man – such as Adolphe Abrahams. Over and over he bemoaned the 'perverted' standards of elite, international-level athletes, and the distance between these 'superathletes' and 'normal men', mirroring earlier concepts of the normal athlete and abnormal freak. Yet Abrahams' protests reveal the fact that a conceptual difference between *normal* man and *abnormal* athlete had already become established. Elsewhere, the provision of special services to athlete and sportsmen give tacit evidence of their 'specialness', from the advanced medical provision in professional sport to the provision for amateurs by medical enthusiasts. So too, while sports injury books paid at least lip-service to the fact that (for example) sprains and strains were not the prerogative of the athlete, they also made note of the 'special' features of the sportsman to argue for his specialist treatment – his eagerness to return to activity, or need for better restorative function than the non-athlete. This differentiation is also present in much of the discussion of fitness and national vitality discussed above; a trend present at the international as well as the national level. The League of Nations' reports between 1937 and 1938 emphasise that physical education was for community and not competition, making clear the division between some sort of lay or civilian participation, and the athlete or sportsman.[124]

Houlihan, in his history of the politics of sport, has suggested that increasing governmental interest in fitness and leisure automatically leads to increased state control of sport.[125] The division between normal man and sportsman show that this connection, while usual, is far from inevitable. A clear counter-example could be the increased interest in physical exercise and fitness at the turn of the century, inspired at least in part by the defeats of the Boer War. Governmental interest here focused almost exclusively on school sports and physical education for the young, and even more specifically on 'scientific' exercise, involving gymnastics and drill rather than any concern with general sports and games.[126]

The complexity of the relationship between elite and organised sport and national 'fitness', however that is to be defined, means that other factors have to coalesce before control of sport becomes a necessity. Indeed, some parts of government, health services, medical professions, and sporting organisations actively avoided any explicit connection between fitness and sport throughout the twentieth century on the grounds that insufficient scientific evidence existed to prove a concrete link (see Chapters 5 and 6). Sports governing bodies and other interested institutions often seemed far more comfortable promoting sport as a social and economic good rather than a health benefit. This, I believe, is evidence of an unresolved ambiguity in the athletic body – the division between healthy 'normal' fitness, and the over-developed, unhealthy, abnormal, specialist, sporting bodies.

Sport cannot therefore be mapped neatly onto physical exercise, school physical education or national fitness schemes, not least because of the important role sportsmen play as entertainers and, increasingly after 1927, as *avatars* for national, political, racial, even gender identities. This role – plus, of course, the increased access to elite medical intervention, a difference between the lay and athletic body that increased over the second half of the twentieth century – distances sports medicine from any mere discussion of fitness, and 'sport' from a close correlation with 'physical exercise'. The distance is also a consequence of outside (international) pressure to improve sporting performances. When the sportsman is no longer just a fit individual, but a national representative, his, and increasingly her, performance on the international stage becomes important as a political tool, and a factor in public confidence and satisfaction in government.

Therefore, a range of influences above and beyond a renewed concern with national fitness led to the increased state, government and other organisational/institutional 'control' of sport. Likewise, a range of related factors came together to allow the concept of sports medicine to emerge as a distinct specialty in Britain. Firstly there was the increased funding of specialisms relevant to sports medicine; this was caused by war, the needs of soldiers, and the formation and activity of the MRC. Secondly, the broadening range and number of 'experts', some produced by the aforementioned medical specialisms, some produced by the international interest in sports medicine, some from the demands by athletes for doctors and auxiliary services (especially at the Olympic Games). Further, these experts were beginning to organise sub-committees, advisory boards and specialist groups. Thirdly, there was the straightforward and intense pressure to improve performance on the international scene. These factors led to a greater (rhetorical if not always real) division between normal and abnormal, layman and athlete. Finally – it is almost inevitable that these forces should also act on sportsmen, who increasingly solicited expert advice, in person, in clinics, from auxiliary medical services, coaches, trainers, team managers or textbooks.

A medically recognised 'special' body; a 'body' of specialists and experts; a 'body' of patients available as a clientele demanding 'specialised' advice and treatment. Thus the scene is set almost requiring the emergence of a single, authoritative 'body' representing medical knowledge in sports and exercise. On 23 June 1952 the first meeting of the organisation to be known as the British Association of Sport and Medicine was held in London. Present were Abrahams as President, Sir Arthur Porritt as Chairman, Dr WS Tegner as honorary secretary and treasurer, and a committee of Brigadier Glyn Hughes, Lt Col Milne, and Mr AE Kendall.[127] The aim of the organisation was stated: 'To promote the study and investigation of all medical aspects of Sport'.[128] The organisation's membership criteria were set:

> Membership will be open to:—
> a) Medical representatives nominated by all national Sporting Bodies.
> b) Medical men and women with a qualification registrable in the United Kingdom who are interested in Sport.
> c) Other scientists with similar interests [who] are eligible for election as honorary members.[129]

Associations were to pay a guinea and individuals 10 shillings each to become members, and adverts were placed in the *Lancet*, the *British Medical Journal*, *Medical World*, and *Medical Press*, and '[i]t was also agreed that the Press Association should be asked for details of Sporting Papers so that the editors of these too can be notified of the formation of the Association'.[130] In the first four months of its existence, 115 people made enquiries regarding membership, and by the time of the first AGM in February 1953, there were 48 paid-up members.[131] The athlete was different; he needed and deserved special treatment. What remained was for his differences to be defined, and for the source of his 'specialist' treatment to be established. These processes will be discussed in the next chapter.

## Notes

1 This pivotal year has also been noted by Roberta Park: RJ Park, 'Cells or Soaring? Historical Reflections on 'Visions' of the Body, Athletics, and Modern Olympism' *Olympika: The International Journal of Olympic Studies* ix (2000), 1–24.

2 S Bailey, *Science in the Service of Physical Education and Sport: The Story of the International Council of Sport Science and Physical Education 1956–1996* (Chichester: John Wiley & Sons, 1996), p.16.

3 Park, 'Cells or Soaring', 13.

4 A Abrahams, 'On the Physiology of violent exercise in relation to the possibility of strain' *Lancet* 211 (1928), 429–35.

5 Anon, 'Sports Doctors' *BMJ* 211 (1928), 365–6.

6 Centre for Sports Science & History, Birmingham University [Hence: CSSH] Archives of the Amateur Athletics Association. XXV.M2, Medical Statistics on 13 Men (Abrahams).

7 AV Hill, *Muscular Movement in Man: The Factors Governing Speed and Recovery from Fatigue* (New York; London: McGraw Hill, 1927); Hill, *Living Machinery* (London: G Bell and Sons Ltd, 1927).

8 CB Heald, *Injuries and Sport. A General Guide for the Practitioner* (Oxford: Oxford University Press, 1931). Other works on the science of exercise included FAM Webster's, *The Science of Athletics* (London: Nicholas Kaye, 1936).

9 Anon, 'Medical News' *Lancet* 231 (1938), 1253.

10 For the increasing importance/popularity of rehabilitation in particular see: MV Lace, *Massage and Medical Gymnastics* (London: J&A Churchill Ltd, 1945 – 3rd edn). On orthopaedics: R Cooter, *Surgery and Society in Peace and War: Orthopaedics and the Organisation of Modern Medicine, 1880–1948* (London: Macmillan, 1993).

11 Physiologists certainly made the connections between war and sport explicit, see: JE Lovelock, 'Physiological and Medical Principles of Training' *Practitioner* 160 (1948), 221–9.

12 This also involved direct propaganda to 'the public', for example thorough radio broadcasts about diet and exercise: 'Towards National Health', *The Listener*, 7 Apr. 1937, 655; much of this work was directed towards school and youth-based physical education, rather than physical exercise. FWW Griffin, *Scientific Basis of Physical Education* (London: Humphrey Milford, Oxford University Press, 1937).

13 The Berlin Olympics of 1936 were the first where accusations of gender fraud were made publicly, with the US team's chaperone, Avery Brundage, suggesting that all 'suspicious' female cases ought to be investigated. Gender testing is discussed in more detail in Chapter 4.

14 This was Augustus Thorndike's, *Athletic Injuries* (Philadelphia: Lea & Febiger, 1938), as cited in AJ Ryan, 'Medical Aspects of Sports' *JAMA* 194 (1965), 173–5. 174.

15 AJ Ryan, 'Standards for physician training in sports medicine' *Clinical Orthopaedics and Related Research* 164 (1982), 13–17. 13.

16 The phrase 'ideal citizens' comes from Heald, where he explicitly suggests that the athlete is a specialist body (as opposed to the 'normal' fit man). Heald is entirely ambiguous about the value of the 'elite' sporting body, suggesting that perhaps its difference from the 'normal' healthy body renders it an undesirable physical state for much of the population. CB Heald, 'Physical Exercise and Sport as Preventives of Disease' *Lancet* 223 (1934), 413–16. 414.

17 Shamateur is a portmanteau word used as a derogatory term referring to sportsmen and women who profess to be amateurs, but who make money from their sporting activity.

18 'Olympic winners are not merely first class, but super class, and these can be no more evolved from ordinary good material than a Caruso could be evolved from an ordinary good tenor. This is of more than academic importance. The craze for Olympic distinction must demand a species of selection directly antagonistic to a general elevation of national athletic ability'. HM Abrahams & A Abrahams, *Training for Athletes* (London: G Bell and Sons Ltd, 1928), p. 175.

19 Anon, 'Injuries and Sport' *BMJ* 2 (1931), 18.

20 See: WGS Pepper, AT Fripp and WE Tanner, 'Injuries to the Professional Association Footballer' *Practitioner* 164 (1950), 298–305. 303.

21 A Abrahams, 'Athletic Training: the Olympic Standard' *Times*, 4 Aug. 1931; Abrahams, 'Berlin and After: The Evolution of Sport' *Times*, 24 Aug. 1936; Abrahams, 'Amateurism in Sport' *Times*, 2 Feb. 1952.

22 Attendance fell again in 1952 to just three masseurs (and the Medical Officer) due to the expense of travelling to Helsinki.

23 Pepper *et al.*, 'Injuries to Professional Football', 298; DF Featherstone, 'Medicine and Sport' *Practitioner* 170 (1953), 299–302.

24 Anon, 'Gleanings: Footballers and National Insurance' *Athletic News*, 17 June 1912.

25 Featherstone, 'Medicine and Sport', 299.

26 Pepper *et al.*, 'Injuries to Professional Football', 298.

27 N Carter, 'Metatarsals and Magic Sponges: English Football and the Development of Sports Medicine' *Journal of Sport History* 31 (2007), 53–73.

28 C Swanston and R Passmore, 'Medical Services in the Small Factory' *Practitioner* 162 (1949), 405–13. By 1951 football club doctors also had a specific handbook: WD Jarvis, *A Medical Handbook for Athletic and Football Club Trainers* (London: Faber and Faber, 1955).

29 Webster, *Science of Athletics*, pp. 263–4.

30 There are four reasons 'why shibboleths remain and prejudices persist'; the lack of research; the 'power of tradition'; the plausibility of faddists' adverts; and the fact that 'men are wary of dropping a system which has suited them reasonably well for another which someone only *says* will lead to better results [original emphasis]'. FAM Webster, *The Science of Athletics* (London: Nicholas Kaye, 1936). 263–4.

31 Holt makes the argument that compulsory physical education for the working classes was generally limited to drill and gymnastics until the 1930s and 1940s, so organised team games were a minority interest. R Holt, *Sport and the British* (Oxford: Clarendon, 1990); see Chapter 3. 'Living In The City: Working Class Communities'.

32 S Sturdy and R Cooter, 'Science, Scientific Management, and the Transformation of Medicine in Britain, c.1870–1950' *History of Science* 36 (1998), 421–66.

33 For a comprehensive account of the work of the Medical Research Council, see A Landsborough Thomson, *Half a Century of Medical Research* (London: HMSO, 1975).

34 PH Newman, JPS Thomson, JM Barnes & TCM Moore, 'A Clinic for Athletic Injuries' *Proceedings of the Royal Society of Medicine* 62 (1969), 939–41.

35 Those who worked in such clinics formed a core of interested enthusiasts; Donald Featherstone, for example, worked as a physiotherapist in Woodard's 'Athletes' Injury Clinic' (see footnote 120, below), went on to take up a variety of posts in sports medicine (Principal of the Athletes' Injury Clinic in Southampton, Physiotherapist to the Southampton Football Club, the Hampshire Cricket Club and the Southampton speedway team), before publishing his own book: DF Featherstone, *Sports Injuries Manual for Trainers and Coaches* (London: Nicholas Kaye, 1954).

36 National Archives [Hence: NA]. FD1/2474. Physical Fitness: Commission on Physical Fitness; Meeting of World Experts 1937–8.

37 Ibid.

38 Ibid.

39 Bailey, Science in the Service, p. 16.

40 G La Cava, 'Editorial: Sports Medicine in Modern Times, A Short Historical Survey', *The Journal of Sports Medicine and Physical Fitness* 3 (1973), 155–8. 155.

41 VN Smodlaka, 'Sports Medicine in the World Today' *JAMA* 205 (1968), 138–9. 138.

42  G Thines & R Zayan, 'FJJ Buytendijk's Contribution to Animal Behaviour: Animal Psychology or Ethology?' *Acta Biotheoretica* XXIV (1975), 86–99.

43  Bailey, *Science in the Service*, p. 16.

44  K Tittel and HG Knuttgen, 'The Development, Objectives and Activities of the International Federation of Sports Medicine (the FIMS)' in A Drix, HG Knuttgen, K Tittel (eds), *The Olympic Book of Sports Medicine: vol 1 of the Encyclopaedia of Sports Medicine* (Oxford, 1988, IOC+the FIMS), pp. 7–12.

45  Park makes the point that German development was inspired by professors rather than physicians, which contributed to the academic early nature of German sports medicine: Park, 'Cells or Soaring?'.

46  JM Hoberman, 'The Early Development of Sports Medicine in Germany' in J Berryman & R Park (eds), *Sport and Exercise Science: Essays in the History of Sports Medicine* (Chicago: University of Illinois Press, 1992), pp. 233–81; F Heiss, 'Sportmedizin im Wandel der Zeiten – 50 Jahre internationaler Sportärzteverband (the FIMS)', *Deutsche Zeitschrift für Sportmedizin* 7 (1978).

47  Hoberman, 'The Early Development', 243.

48  Amsterdam Olympic Committee, *The Official Report of the IXth Olympiad, Amsterdam, 1928* (Amsterdam: Olympic Committee of the Amsterdam Olympic Games, 1928), pp. 948–51.

49  Amsterdam Olympic Committee, *The Official Report of the Amsterdam Olympiad*.

50  Unless otherwise stated, the details of provision come from: LA Olympic Committee, *The Games of the Xth Olympiad, Los Angeles 1932, Official Report* (Los Angeles: Olympic Committee of the Los Angeles Olympic Games, 1932), p. 185.

51  Ibid., p. 189.

52  Ibid., p. 194.

53  The British doctors were WV Chalmers Francis MD and George Martin MD. The complete list of medical advisers and support staff in the official report is four pages long.

54  Unless otherwise stated, the details of provision come from: Berlin Olympic Committee, *The Official Report of the XIth Olympiad, Berlin* (Berlin: Olympic Committee of the Berlin Olympic Games, 1936).

55  See also a report in the *BMJ*, about a bureau 'to be set up to allow medical men there to learn about the various medical institutions and arrangements in Berlin' as part of the Congress on Sports Medicine (the FIMS) run concurrently with the Olympics. Anon 'Medical News' *BMJ* 2(1936), 107.

56  London Olympic Committee, *The Official Report of the Organising Committee for the XIV Olympiad* (London: The Organising Committee for the XIV Olympiad, 1948).

57  Archives of the British Olympic Association. 1948 Games (Organizing Committee) Medical Committee 1946–8 [Hence: Minutes of the Medical Committee, 1948]; First Meeting of the Medical General Committee of the Organising Committee for XIV Olympiad London 10 Oct. 1946

58  London Olympic Committee, *Official Report 1948*, p. 185.

59  Minutes of the Medical Committee, 1948. 26 Feb. 1947.

60  Minutes of the Medical Committee, 1948. 9 Apr. 1948.

61  London Olympic Committee, *Official Report 1948*, p. 190.

62  Ibid., p. 191.

63  Ibid., p. 192.

64  'The basins were in many cases disregarded by the athletes, who stepped across them, so that their actual value was questionable', Berlin Olympic Committee, *Official Report 1936*, p. 464.

65  'Briefly, Dybowska and Dybowski and Kohlrausch made anthropometric and functional capacity measurements; Thörner studied haematology at rest; Bramwell and Ellis, Deutsch, Herxheimer, Hoogerwerf, Bürger *et al.* investigated various cardiovascular aspects; Hüntermuller studied the immune system; while Shenk and Craemer and Snapper and Grünbaum considered blood and urine biochemistry. In addition, Best and Partridge and Messerli (not official members of this investigative team) respectively, measured blood glucose levels and provided a description of the actual marathon race'. MB Maron & SM Horvath, 'The Marathon: a History and Review of the Literature' *Medicine and Science in Sports* 10 (1978), 137–50. 139. See also: CH Best & RC Partridge, 'Observations on Olympic Athletes' *Proceedings of the Royal Society of London, Series B* 105 (1929), 323–32; C Bramwell & R Ellis, 'Clinical Observations on Olympic athletes' *Arbeitsphysiologie* 1 (1928), 51–60.

66  LA Olympic Committee, *Official Report 1932*.

67  Bramwell & Ellis, 'Clinical Observations'. Examinations were also made of some auxiliary staff, such as team managers. HM Abrahams (ed.), *The Official Report of the IXth Olympiad, Amsterdam, 1928*, (London: British Olympic Association, 1948), pp. 265–6.

68  A Abrahams, 'Boat-Race Crews: Tests of Physical Fitness' *Times*, 31 Mar. 1933.

69  Ibid.

70  A Abrahams, 'Physical Exercise, its Clinical Association' *Lancet* 257 (1951), 1133–7. 1136.

71  A Abrahams, 'Athletic Training: the Olympic Standard' *Times*, 4 Aug. 1931; Abrahams, 'Olympic Games; Factors in Success or Failure; The British Showing' *Times*, 13 Aug. 1948; Abrahams, 'Athletic Talent at Helsinki' *Times*, 31 Jul. 1952.

72  Women's marathon was not introduced into the Olympic programme until 1984, so the gender pronoun is correct.

73  Bramwell and Ellis examined sprinters, middle- and long-distance runners, and marathoners, and their 'object in so doing [was] to find out whether there is any obvious difference in so far as the cardiovascular mechanism is concerned, between these different groups'. Bramwell and Ellis, 'Clinical Observations', pp. 51–2.

74  A fact recognised by contemporaries, see: 'The Science of Exercise' *Lancet* 219 (1932), 988. This editorial cites Abrahams and Hill as honourable exceptions

to the fact that in Britain 'interest in the theoretical side of athletics has not been so universal as in other countries'.

75  VO$_2$max, expressed in litres of oxygen per minute (or more recently in millilitres of oxygen per kilogramme of body weight), is intended as an absolute measure of the maximum capacity of an individual to utilise inspired oxygen; it is usually regarded as a measurement indicating 'fitness', especially for endurance sports.

76  Hill, Muscular Movement in Man, p. 3.

77  After Hill in 1922, Nobel Prizes for Medicine or Physiology were awarded in sports medicine-relevant areas for the refinement of the electrocardiogram in 1924, for exercise-relevant studies of respiration in 1931 and 1938, the nervous system in 1932 and 1936, and glycogen metabolism in 1947.

78  Abrahams bemoaned athletes' keenness to use modern 'faddist' or 'fashionable' medical interventions, particularly doping with vitamins. A Abrahams 'Diet and Physique' Practitioner 155 (1945), 370–7.

79  A Abrahams, 'Arris and Gale Lecture, on the physiology of Violent Exercise in Relation to the Possibility of Strain' Lancet 211 (1928), 429–35. Dr Heald also drew on the work of Hill in writing Sports Injuries (published in 1931).

80  J Hoberman, Mortal Engines: The Science of Performance and the Dehumanization of Sport (New Jersey: Blackburn Press, 1992), pp. 72–6.

81  Hoberman, Mortal Engines; Hoberman, Testosterone Dreams. Rejuvenation, Aphrodisia, Doping (Berkeley; LA; London: University of California Press, 2005). see also D Hamilton, The Monkey Gland Affair (London: Chatto and Windus, 1986).

82  Anon, 'Gland Final' Daily Mirror, 21 Jul. 1978, 20.

83  'The practice of giving gland treatment to footballers is now growing more widespread than was ever expected, and the day is not far away when 'tired' players in nearly every club in the country will be brought back to form with these special courses.' J Thompson, 'John Thompson's Sportfolios – Why They Go On With Glands' Daily Mirror, 16 Sept. 1938.

84  Anon, 'The Unnatural Athlete' Lancet 234 (1939), 211.

85  Anon, 'Attack on Glands', Daily Mirror 8 Mar. 1939.

86  See in particular P Dimeo, A History of Drug Use in Sport, 1875–1976, Beyond Good and Evil (London: Routledge, 2007) and R Beamish and I Ritchie, 'From Fixed Capacities to Performance-Enhancing Substances' Sport in History 25 (2005), 412–33.

87  'This term ['athlete's heart'], if legitimately employed, would apply to a heart of superior contractility particularly efficient for the circulatory demands of athletic feats and of violent exercise generally'. A Abrahams, 'Physical Exercise – its clinical application' Lancet 257 (1951), 1133–7.

88  The kidney had also been part of the ab/normal debate in the early twentieth century, with regard to albinuria (protein in the urine, normally symptomatic of kidney malfunction or damage). In reflection of the Athlete's Heart story, the presence of albumin in the urine was originally considered a danger sign (leading to clinicians recommending the permanent cessation of exercise)

until work in 1907 instead promoted the idea that athletic 'pseudonephritis' was a non-pathological clinical oddity. The Athlete's Kidney was reinvented as a genuine pathological presentation only after 1960. W Collier, 'The Kidney and Exercise' *Transactions of the Medical Society of London* 30 (1907), 75; Anon 'Annotations: The Kidney and Exercise' *Lancet* 233 (1939), 939–40; KD Gardener, 'Athletic Nephritis: Pseudo and Real' *Annals of Internal Medicine* 75 (1971), 966.

89 Most obviously, tennis elbow: Anon, 'Royal Society of Medicine: Orthopaedics – Tennis Elbow' *Lancet* 215 (1929), 1257–8; T Marlin, 'Treatment of "Tennis Elbow" with some Observations on Joint Manipulation' *Lancet* 215 (1930), 509–11; 'Tennis Elbow' *Lancet* 215 (1930), 660; 'Tennis Elbow' *Practitioner* 164 (1950), 293–7.

90 Anon, 'Injuries and sport, Book Review' *Lancet* 218 (1931), 638–9.

91 Heald, 'Physical Exercise and Sport'.

92 Ibid.

93 What is also notable is the long list of 'sporting injuries' with distinctive names – Heald includes Bowler's arm, Golfer's Shoulder, Football Shoulder, Rider's Strain, Games Knee and Tennis Leg along with the more familiar Tennis Elbow and Athlete's Foot. Clearly these injuries/conditions had been present as named clinical entities before 1931. Tucker adds the terms Rugby Shoulder, Golfer's Wrist and Wicket Keepers' Finger to the list of specially named sports injuries. A study of the origins of so-called 'sports injuries' would be informative. Heald, *Injuries and Sport*. WE Tucker, 'Athletic Injuries' in H Rolleston (ed.) *The British Encyclopaedia of Medical Practice – Volume II* (London, Butterworth, 1936), pp. 225–38.

94 Just as examples – see: SS Knight, *Fitness and Injury in Sport* (London: Skeffington, 1952); Lovelock, 'Physiotherapy and the Athlete'; Lovelock, 'Physiological and Medical Principles of Training'; Abrahams, 'Physical Exercise: its Clinical Association'; WE Tucker, 'Cricketing Injuries' *Practitioner* 162 (1949), 496–501; Pepper *et al.*, 'Injuries to the Professional Association Footballer', 427. See also a series of articles in the *BMJ* on skiing: 1 (1951), 401–2, 586, 761–2.

95 And, of course, sportsmen themselves continued to turn to 'science' to give them an edge, as evidenced by the advertising schemes of vitamin extracts, Oxo and Bovril, Dextrosol, etc. See for example the adverts (including those for Horlicks, 'Glucose, lifes [sic] vital force', and Elliman's Embrocation) at the back of FAM Webster & JA Heys, *Athletic Training for Men and Boys: A Comprehensive System of Training Tables for all Events* (London: Shaw, 1933).

96 John Welshman, 'Only Connect: The History of Sport, Medicine and Society' *International Journal of the History of Sport* 15 (1998), 1–21; KG Sheard, ''Brutal and Degrading': The Medical Profession and Boxing, 1838–1984' *International Journal of the History of Sport* 15 (1998), 74–102.

97 And also interest in the fit, young, male, athlete-soldier's body – boxing after all was widely used as physical training in the British Armed Forces. CE Winterstein, 'Head Injuries Attributable to Boxing' *Lancet* 230 (1937),

719–20; E Jokl, *The Medical Aspects of Boxing* (Pretoria; JL Van Schaik Ltd, 1941); JA Milspaugh, 'Boxing and Parkinsonism' *Practitioner* 2 (1948), 513; EW Busse & AJ Silverman, 'Electroencephalographic Changes in Professional Boxers' *JAMA* 120 (1952), 1522–5. It is also worth noting that some researchers saw the value of boxers as guinea-pigs, in the same way that other scientists and doctors had used athletes and sporting events – as Winterstein (cited above) writes: 'boxing [is] a model experiment for the study of traumatic head injury'. Winterstein, 'Head Injuries', 719.

98 Welshman, 'Only Connect', 8.

99 See J Anderson, "Turned into Taxpayers': Paraplegia, Rehabilitation and Sport at Stoke Mandeville, 1944–56, *Journal of Contemporary History* 38 (2003), 461–75; J Scruton, *Stoke Mandeville – Road to the Paralympics* (Aylesbury: Peterhouse, 1998).

100 L Guttman, 'Significance of Sport in Rehabilitation of Spinal Paraplegics and Tetraplegics' *JAMA* 236 (1976), 195–7. 195.

101 Ibid., 196.

102 For earlier European interventions, see M Atherton, 'Sport in the British Deaf Community' *Sport in History* 27 (2007), 276–92; D Séguillon, 'The Origins and Consequences of the First World Games for the Deaf: Paris, 1924' *International Journal of the History of Sport* 19 (2002), 119–32.

103 Scruton, *Stoke Mandeville*, p. 290.

104 S Bailey, *Athlete First: A History of the Paralympic Movement* (Chichester: John Wiley & Sons, 2008).

105 These reactions were not limited to the UK. See the account of physical training programmes in inter-war North America: RE Johnson 'Applied Physiology' *Annual Review of Physiology* 8 (1946), 535–8.

106 For example, experiments on the use of vitamins in the improvement of physical performance: Abrahams, 'Physical Exercise, its Clinical Association', 1135. This was particularly problematic for the 1948 London Olympics, where matters of food allowance became highly controversial.

107 Landsborough Thomson, *Half a Century of Medical Research*. Vol. I Part I.

108 Ibid. Vol. II, 137–61.

109 Of relevance too was the Department of the Physiology of Sex Hormones, founded in 1932.

110 Anon, 'Medical Research Council Report for 1937–8' *Lancet* 239 (1939), 525; Landsborough Thomson, *Half a Century of Medical Research*. Vol II, 95.

111 Abrahams, 'Physical Exercise', 1136–7.

112 [NA] ED113/49. *Medical Sub-committee on the desirability of athletics for Women and Girls; Medical Sub-committee on the Criteria of Fitness*. M(38)5. National Advisory Committee for Physical Training and Recreation Medical Committee, 15 June 1939.

113 Ibid. MWG(39)4. *Minutes of the Medical Sub-Committee on the Desirability of Athletics for Women and Girls*. 31 May 1939.

114 Ibid. MWG(39)2. 22 Mar. 1939.

115 A Abrahams, 'Tests for Athletic Efficiency' *Lancet* 234 (1939), 309–12.

116 EP Cathcart, 'Physiological approach to fitness' *BMJ* 2 (1938), 273–6. 273. Although published in a medical journal, this is an outline of the definition of fitness produced by the NFC.

117 Johnson, 'Applied Physiology'.

118 These distinctions are often controversial; see the debate in the letters page of the *Lancet* in November 1937, between Abrahams, Cecil Flemming, Barcroft and others about the definition of the word 'fitness'; *Lancet* 230 (1937), 1140–2, 1217, 1276–7.

119 RS Woods, 'Physical Medicine' *Practitioner* 2 (1943), 263–70. 267. Physical Medicine developed as a specialty directly from the need to treat physically injured military personnel during the World War II.

120 Most sources claim that the Sports Clinic at Middlesex hospital was founded in 1948 by Dr Ben Woodard (Dr Christopher Roy 'Ben' Woodard), who was involved with the AAA and was a consultant to the British Olympic Team in 1948 and 1952. Woodard was apparently employed as an 'Accident Officer' by the Middlesex. The Middlesex Hospital records certainly confirm the setting up of an Accident Service to provide orthopaedic services, but there is no record of a Dr Woodard, or of a sports clinic in what remains of the 1948 reports and minutes. University College London NHS Foundation Trust Archives. *Minutes of the Board of Governors (Middlesex Hospital) Jul 1946–Jun 1948*; Board meeting 18 Sep. 1946 [setting up of Accident Service]. See also: Newman *et al.* 'A Clinic for Athletic Injuries'. C Woodard, *Sports Injuries: Prevention and Active treatment* (Max Parrish: London, 1954).

121 Lovelock, 'Physiotherapy and the Athlete', 227.

122 FS Cooksey, 'Physical Medicine' *Practitioner* 155 (1945), 300–5.

123 SG Jones, 'State Intervention in Sport and Leisure in Britain between the Wars' *Journal of Contemporary History* 22 (1987), 163–82.

124 [NA] FD1/2474. Physical Fitness: Commission on Physical Fitness; Meeting of World Experts 1937–8.

125 B Houlihan, *The Government and Politics of Sport* (London: Routledge, 1991).

126 V Heggie, "Lies, Damn Lies and Manchester's Recruiting Statistics: Degeneration as an "Urban Legend" in Victorian and Edwardian Britain' *Journal of the History of Medicine and Allied Sciences*, 63 (2008), 178–216.

127 Kenneth Sandilands ('Sandy') Duncan (see Chapter 4) was invited but could not attend. British Association of Sport and Exercise Medicine Archives [Hence: BAS(E)M]. *Minutes of the Executive Committee*. 23 Jun. 1952.

128 Ibid.

129 Ibid.

130 Ibid; A Abrahams and AE Porritt, 'Sport and Medicine' *Lancet* 260 (1952), 90; A Abrahams and AE Porritt, 'Sport and Medicine' *BMJ* 2 (1952), 98.

131 [BAS(E)M] Minutes of the Executive Committee. 13 Oct. 1952.

## Box 4. Archibald Vivian Hill (1886–1977)

Archibald Vivian Hill was the UK's leading exercise physiologist in the twentieth century. Educated in Natural Sciences and Physiology at Trinity College, Cambridge, Hill has been described as a 'professional schoolboy of sport', funding his own education through scholarships.[1] His research career started at Trinity College, Cambridge, and in the laboratory of the editor of *The Journal of Physiology*, and included a stint in Tübingen in Germany in 1911. In wartime he worked on anti-aircraft technology, before returning to physiology with a chair in the discipline at Manchester University (1920–23). Hill left for a professorship at University College London just before it was announced that he was to win the 1922 Nobel Prize for his work on 'the conversion of glycogen to lactic acid and its oxidative resynthesis during recovery'.[2] It would be impossible to list all of Hill's 'discoveries' or notable publications; an edited list gives an idea of the significance of his work: 'oxygen debt'; $VO_2Max$; lactic acid and anaerobic exercise; how to establish the role of ATP in muscle metabolism; heat production in nerves.

Hill was widely active outside the laboratory, perhaps most notably on the Academic Assistance Council which relocated Jewish scientists to the USA and UK. As a selection – he was also secretary of the Royal Society (1935–45), Scientific Advisor to the Government of India (1943–44), Independent MP for Cambridge (1940–45), Trustee of the British Museum (1947–63) and President of the British Association for the Advancement of Science (1952).[1]

[1] Anon 'AV Hill – Obituary' *BMJ* 2 (1977), 51.
[2] E Jokl, 'Professor AV Hill, a Personal Tribute' *Journal of Sports Medicine and Physical Fitness* 20 (1980), 465–8.
  See also: LA Reynolds and EM Tansey (eds), *The Development of Sports Medicine in Twentieth Century Britain* (London: Wellcome Trust, 2009), p. 119.

---

### Box 5. Arthur Espie Porritt (1900–94)

Arthur Espie Porritt became the Lord Porritt with the awarding of a Baronetcy (of Wanganiu and Hampstead) in 1973. The New Zealand-born surgeon came to the UK as a Rhodes Scholar at Magdalen College, Oxford, and completed his training at St Mary's Hospital, London. As was the case with many of the early sports medicine practitioners, Porritt had a personal interest in sport, achieving international success in athletics. He held records for 100 and 220 yards hurdles at Oxford, was Captain of the New Zealand Olympic team in 1924 and 1928 (and Manager in Berlin in 1936) and took Olympic Bronze for the 100m in 1924.[1]

Porritt was active in many formal medical organisations, including the British Medical Association (President 1960–61), the Royal College of Surgeons (President 1960–63), and the Royal School of Medicine (President 1966–67). With respect to sports medicine, he sat on the British Olympic Council, and the International Olympic Committee, as well as the British Empire and Commonwealth Games Federation, BAS(E)M and the Institute of Sports Medicine. Some of his direct influence in the UK was interrupted by his appointment as Governor General of New Zealand from 1967–72.[2]

[1] DF Gerrard, 'The Lord Porritt – Obituary' *BJSM* 28 (1994), 77–8.
[2] P Sperryn, 'The Lord Porrit – Obituary' *BJSM* 28 (1994), 78.
   See also in LA Reynolds and EM Tansey (eds), *The Development of Sports Medicine in Twentieth Century Britain* (London: Wellcome Trust, 2009), p.126.

---

## Box 6. The Central Council of Physical Recreation (CCPR)

The CCPR was founded in 1935 as the Central Council of Recreative Physical Training. Many influences led to its formation, specifically the 'poor conditions of youth', and the success of similar movements overseas, such as the rise of the Hitler Youth.[1] As Evans has suggested in his 'official' history of the CCPR, 'four factors created a favourable climate' for the CCPR, increased interest in physical education, fears about national health, rising unemployment and 'a growing recognition on the part of voluntary bodies which had hitherto worked in isolation that they needed the additional strength that could come from co-operation'.[2] Originally membership was ad hoc and thus limited to enthusiasts, most inspired by the Minister of Health, Sir Hilton Young who, at a dinner of the British Medical Association, encouraged the formation of such an organisation. But this system 'gave way to a system of affiliation by national organisations'.[1]

The CCPR benefited from the Physical Training and Recreation Act in 1937, and the interest in physical education which resulted, and was largely funded by grants from the Ministry of Education. As such, it specialised in the funding of training schemes for coaches and other sports professionals, and was involved with the founding of Britain's Sports Centre at Bisham Abbey. Until the 1960s it was the 'go to' body for advice and professional opinion on training and sports schemes, especially for young people.

It was the CCPR which initiated the Wolfenden Report (1960–61 – See Chapter 4), which led to a significant change for the organisation. The CCPR worked with, in parallel, and represented on, the committees of the resultant Sports Council, to which it handed over its assets in 1972, recognising the Sports Council as a central administrative body. The Council gives financial support to the CCPR, which is now intended as a representative body for sports that is independent of government.[3]

[1] B Houlihan, *The Government and Politics of Sport* (London: Routledge, 1991).
[2] HJ Evans, *Service to Sport: the story of the CCPR, 1937 – 1975* (London: Pelham (In Assoc with the Sports Council), 1974).
[3] [CSSH] Archives of the Sports Council. *Minutes of the Sports Council.* Various.

# 4

# Making champions: boundaries, 1953–70

By 1953 the athlete and the non-athlete were different. Significantly, athletes had different needs as patients as well as being medically and physiologically distinct. The athlete, Adolphe Abrahams insisted, 'regarded himself as a privileged person' in terms of medical treatment.[1] He did not always get the specialist treatment he desired, but through the period considered in this chapter his opportunity to be cared for by people with specific experience in managing sportspeople was improving. This chapter opens with the first meetings of BAS(E)M, a society dedicated to the collation and provision of specialist sports medicine advice, and it closes in 1970 with the Sports Council initiating a study into the feasibility of using taxpayers' money to fund sports injuries clinics for the general public.

The intervening years saw a proliferation of organisations related to sports medicine ; after BAS(E)M in 1953 came the British Olympic Association's Medical Committee (1959), the Institute of Sports Medicine (1963), the Sports Council's Research and Statistics Committee (1965), and other specialist organisations.[2] As a consequence this chapter spends more time discussing institutions and their activities than has been the case for previous chapters. The work of these organisations, how they conceptualised their roles, tends to highlight the changed nature of the athletic body in this time period. Interest in general fitness, in physical education, in the 'health of the nation' was stripped away, leaving a clear concentration on the elite, ab- or super-normal athletic body. This was even the case for the Sports Council, despite the fact that this organisation was set up as a response to the Wolfenden Committee on Sport (f.1957) which had explicitly aimed to consider sport as a means to 'promo[te] the general welfare of the community'.[3]

The key issue for this chapter is boundary-setting. Firstly, and most practically, sports medicine was being institutionalised in small professional organisations, which carefully policed their own boundaries. They were filled with members who regarded themselves, and were sometimes recognised by outside groups, as having uncommon and specialised knowledge. While these organisations were partly interested in deciding who was and who was not an expert in sports medicine, they were also particularly focused on defining the bodies of sports medicine's patients. So secondly, boundaries were being drawn around the athletic body. Having established athletes as different, the question to be answered was *how* different? Different in what ways? If athletes were no longer normal, what was 'normal' for the athlete?

A great deal of the work of these new sports medicine organisations seems to be focused on finding ways to investigate and then define the athletic body – and examples of such activity will form the bulk of the chapter to follow. In particular we see attempts to establish formal systems and locations for experimental research in sports medicine (including, but not limited to, exercise physiology). Laboratory and clinic overlapped in the many surveys and epidemiological studies which also characterise sports medicine in the 1950s and 1960s; these are clear attempts to find statistical measures which define and explain the athletic body. They are also, in the case of the injuries surveys which will be discussed below, an attempt to prove that there was a distinct patient population that desired and deserved specialist sports medicine facilities and treatment.

In the middle of the twentieth century we also see, quite dramatically on the world stage, the practical application of these boundaries of normality and abnormality. Three issues dominate international sports medicine between 1953 and 1970; dope tests, gender tests and (at a distance) the issue of competition at altitude. All of these are issues which are ostensibly about 'fair competition', but which absolutely require rigorous – sometimes chemical – definitions of the athletic body. To decide how much of a particular hormone an athlete may have in their blood sample before they are disqualified sports organisations require not just 'normal' standards, but standards specifically tailored for sports men and women, whose physiology may significantly differ from that of the 'man on the street'. Dope and gender tests also cut the other way – they illustrate specifically that the athlete is *different*. Substances (caffeine, cough medicine) which are at worst harmless, and at best possibly curative, in the 'normal' body now become dangerous and illegitimate in the body of the athlete. It became possible for someone to be born and live as a woman, even bear children, and still not count as 'female' for the purpose of international sport.[4] Even a category as apparently basic as male/female has different boundaries when applied to the athletic body.

It is no coincidence that just as these issues of definition and disqualification became central in elite sports, so we see a proliferation of experts who were able to police these boundaries. These trends are self-feeding; increased demand increases funding which increases research opportunities which increases interest in the field. The more the athletic body was found to be different the more it needed to be studied. As Guiseppe La Cava, Secretary of FIMS, wrote in 1960, much had been discovered about the cardiovascular system of the athlete, but comparatively little was known about 'for instance . . . the endocrine system and . . . the antitoxic functions'.[5] What was being sought was the standardised athlete, deviations from which could lead to disqualification or disadvantage. It was this standardised athlete who would be used to decide if environmental conditions suited or harmed athletic performance, if this or that chromosomal abnormality precluded competing in women's events. It was in the best interest of all nations to ensure that this standardised athlete most closely matched their own ideals; and if biomedicine was going to be used to test this body, biomedicine needed to be mobilised to define and then protect it.

## Surveying the athletic body

Before turning more specifically to the whens, wheres and whos of sports medicine in Britain in this time period, we should consider one final kind of boundary-setting, that of the ultimate physical limits of human performance. The mid-1950s were an important period for physical limits, with Tenzing Norgay and Edmund Hillary's ascent of Everest in 1953, followed in 1954 by Bannister's sub-four-minute mile.[6] These achievements contrasted with a British sporting experience between 1953 and 1970 which was, with notable exceptions (Everest, Bannister, and the 1966 World Cup in particular) relatively disappointing. The Olympic medal tally fell progressively and there was the occasional unusually humiliating sporting defeat, such as the 5–3 victory of the Hungarian football team over England in 1953. This experience is reflective of a much more competitive international sporting scene, one in which both sides of the Cold War regarded sport as yet another proving ground for their particular social systems and political ideologies.[7]

Attempts to define *how* fast, *how* high, *how* strong in relation to the athletic body took place in small university laboratories, in corners of NHS hospitals given over to temporary athletic clinics, in the research facilities of the Medical Research Council (often co-sponsored by the Sports Council or directed by BAS(E)M members), and in some cases in exotic locations. from Mexico to St Moritz. Much of this activity we must consider sports science rather than explicitly sports medicine; but as a new site of practice the laboratory went from strength to strength between 1953 and 1970. Perhaps the best symbol of British sports medicine in the mid-century is the mobile laboratory at Crystal Palace, set up in 1967, and eventually becoming a permanent laboratory with meeting rooms in 1972.

This laboratory was founded by the Sports Council, a new player in sports medicine from 1965. The Council had been created as a direct result of the recommendations of the Wolfenden Committee on Sport, which itself had been initiated in 1957 by the Central Council of Physical Recreation (in co-operation with the Scottish CPR). Chaired by Sir John Wolfenden (1906–85), among the eight members of the Committee representing interests from politics, sports and physical education, was Sir Arthur Porritt. The aims of the Committee, were to '[e]xamine the factors affecting the development of games, sports and outdoor activities' and to make recommendations for change which would ensure 'that these activities may play their full part in promoting the general welfare of the community'.[8] Much of the Wolfenden Committee's Report, published in 1960, considered aspects of participation and access to facilities.[9] Sports medicine is minimally considered, being mentioned in passing in a single paragraph, although the likelihood that sport is healthy is repeated at several points.[10] The Committee's major recommendation was the founding of a 'Sports Development Council' (structured like the Arts Council), independent of government and funded 'directly by the Treasury' which could give grants to applicants, such as the BOA or the various national governing bodies of sport.[11] This money should also be used, the Report suggests, to fund sports medicine through bodies like BAS(E)M, 'the Consultant Medical Panel of the CCPR, the Ergonomics Society, certain branches of the [MRC] and the Medical Officers of the Governing Bodies of sport'.[12]

The Sports Council is technically the 'Advisory Sports Council' for the period 1965–72, to distinguish it from the executive body it became with a reorganisation and reform in 1972. (Since the Council refers to itself as simply the 'Sports Council' in most of its own records before and after 1972 I have used that term consistently throughout this book). From its formation in 1965 this Council showed much more interest in exercise science and sports medicine than the Wolfenden Committee had done. For example, it quickly expressed an interest in establishing a 'permanent centre for sports medicine research', which became the first point on the agenda of its Research and Statistics Committee, and representatives of this committee approached the Medical Research Council (not, interestingly, the British Olympic Association or BAS(E)M) for advice and co-operation.[13] The MRC were keen to have a biomechanical laboratory available for their researchers, but were wary about being drawn into research that was too sports-specific. For them the athlete was no longer the all-round useful guinea pig, and was 'but one approach to the field of human physiology'.[14]

This is not to suggest that the MRC was disinterested in exercise physiology, or in probing the special physiology of the athlete. By 1963 its own list of 'sports related' research included studies of body fat in channel swimmers, physiological testing at the 1958 British Empire and Commonwealth Games in Cardiff, research into the ergonomics of weight-lifting and pole-vaulting, some anthropometric surveys at the 1960 Rome Olympiad, acclimatisation and respiration studies on mountaineers, and a study of golfers.[15] That two of these research projects took place at major international sporting events is fairly representative of research trends in sports medicine at mid-century. The Olympics had been the site of some physiological work from 1928 onwards, and the Commonwealth Games provided a similar opportunity from 1930.

Some of these research projects were clinical studies, and some were attempts to find physical limits for human bodies, but many others were focused on gathering statistical information about the athletic body. As such they were part of the efforts to define this new clinical entity (and, after all, where better to find it than at such large gatherings of supernormal physiques?). These surveys were not limited to Britain; in 1963 the FIMS-inspired 'Olympic Medical Archives' scheme was launched to gather physiological data about Olympic athletes specifically to 'establish adult norms for the highest level of physical fitness' (see Box 7).[16] This short-lived scheme was also intended to trace the after-histories of elite athletes, to track the effect of sporting excellence on morbidity and mortality.

Surveys were also being designed in Britain to demonstrate that athletes were a distinct patient group, as well as establishing them as a discrete physiological type. Sports injury/disease surveys were used to demonstrate that there was a specific clinical need for sports medicine that was not being fulfilled by the NHS. In the late 1960s the Sports Council funded a major injuries survey, which was explicitly for the purpose of investigating the need for specialist medical provision; meanwhile BAS(E)M collaborated with the Coroners' Society in 1969 to produce a 'Sports Mortality Survey'.[17]

One of the largest injuries surveys was carried out by Drs H Evans Robson (1923–92) and JGP Williams (see Box 9). Robson and Williams used a self-reporting system, asking in the popular athletics press (e.g. *Athletics Weekly*) for athletes who had sustained injuries between August 1959 and August 1960 to fill in and return a questionnaire.[18] They also sent out surveys to 'many athletes, coaches and club secretaries' and

> to all kinds of sports men and games players and their clubs throughout the length and breadth of the country in the most complete enquiry ever attempted into the epidemiology of sports injuries in Britain.[19]

The survey work was supported by Loughborough Training College where Robson was a lecturer in anatomy and physiology. University and college laboratories were key parts of sports medicine work in the second half of the twentieth century, although they tended to approach sports medicine from different directions (e.g. as offshoots of the medical school, or of the exercise physiology laboratories).[20]

Surveys such as Williams' and Robson's beg the question of whether the athletic body is 'different' or whether sports injuries can be treated as a distinct category of disability; the survey itself *presupposes* that this is the case. Williams, as the author of the first book in English with the phrase 'sports medicine' in the title, said as much explicitly in his seminal text of 1962:

> [t]he intensity and diversity of modern competitive sport ... and the increased knowledge and experience of the Physical Educationist has resulted in the emergence from the general mass of the population of a *new type of person – the trained athlete*. Whether amateur or professional, he is as different physiologically and psychologically from 'the man in the street' as is the chronic invalid [my emphasis].[21]

Williams' book is important, not just because of his explicit statement of the special needs of the athlete, but also because it is representative of one further trend in sports medicine in Britain, and across the world, in the 1950s and 1960s – the codification of rules and regulations.

Rules are most obviously connected with issues of enhancement in sport – drug regulations, gender tests and so on, but they also began to be codified with regard to mainstream treatment – away from the laboratory now, and into the field and the clinic. By 1953 the standard advised treatment for the most common sports injuries had reached a state which in many cases would be recognisable to twenty-first-century sports medicine (rest, heat and cold, graduated return to activity, etc.) While Heald's *Injuries in Sport* and similar books were already available, Williams' *Sports Medicine* was the first text to attempt a synthetic summary of sports medicine practice in its entirety.[22] The holistic conceptualisation of sports medicine, interdisciplinary and multi-practitioner, is well illustrated by *Sports Medicine*. Contributors to the volume include: a senior registrar in orthopaedics; a consultant physician; a lecturer in anatomy and physiology; a registrar in dermatology; and the senior coach of the AAA (a man without any formal medical qualifications). Information about sports medicine also continued to be available, as it had been since the early 1900s, to the literate layman through texts aimed at the athlete himself.[23]

Despite the increasing codification and standardisation of treatment it is clear that some (possibly even most) sports medicine practice disappointed both its patients and its experts. For example, although the value of exercise instead of rest for sprains and strains had been promoted for over 50 years (see Chapter 2), some practitioners still immobilised their patients in plaster rather than, or instead of, using a physiotherapist. Likewise, even as sports organisations increased their recommendations and requirements for medical coverage at sporting events, these were still often a *desired* level of provision rather than reflecting the reality of sports medicine and sports injury experience more generally.[24] The defining of the athletic body also required the reconstruction of some extant rules, due to the intervention of medical or scientific experts. A good example would be the arrangements for managing marathons in the late 1950s; the Amateur Athletics Association found itself under pressure not just from medical professionals but also its own athlete members to change its rules and allow more refreshment stations along the course of marathons. The Medical Officer of the Road Runner's Club, Dr Lee, argued not only that there should be more stations, but also that recent research suggested that salted drinks should be provided rather than just water.[25]

During the 1950s and 1960s, medical intervention and supervision on the field was increasingly regulated. Although not always obligatory, trainers and coaches involved with professional Association Football clubs were more likely to undertake formal first-aid and physiotherapeutic training; in professional boxing the attendance of doctors at every bout was already mandatory.[26] By 1957 the official AAA Handbook carried clear rules about medical provision for competitive events, including requirements for 'first aid, [a] Medical Officer, a link with the local hospital, transport, and a sealed surgical drum', and by 1969 it appears that most sports governing bodies had appointed official medical officers or advisors.[27] (The regularisation of medical provision at the international level is discussed in more detail below, in connection with the Olympics).

### Sex and drugs

One outstanding feature of international sports medicine at the mid-century is the introduction of gender and drug testing. Both of these activities are explicitly about constructing 'normality' for athletes; both are also often associated with the increasing success (and thus suspicion) of, sportsmen and women from the Eastern Bloc.[28] In fact, gender testing of one sort or another had been in place since at least 1936, when the supporters of Polish runner Stella Walsh, whose tragic death opened this book, accused the American sprinter Helen Stephens of being a man.[29] The German authorities carried out an unspecified check and declared Stephens a woman, and therefore eligible for the gold, while Walsh took silver.[30] By 1946 the International Amateur Athletics Association required a femininity certificate for all women competitors (rule 17 paragraph 3).[31]

*Pace* the traditional 'cold war' stories it was actually a British and a Czechoslovakian athlete who first inspired concern about policing the boundaries of gender in international sport. The former, Mary Louise Edith Weston, had been national javelin champion and international shot put champion, and had 'a series of operations in Charing Cross hospital', in 1936, emerging as Mr Mark Watson and changing career from athlete to masseur.[32] The Czech runner, Zdenka Koubkova, changed sex in 1934. It was Koubkova and Weston's case that led the chaperone of the American Olympic Team to begin a campaign for formal sex testing in the late 1930s.[33]

Weston's story is usually left out of accounts of gender testing, perhaps because of the dominance of the Cold War as an explanatory paradigm.[34] In fact, instead of being a phenomenon of the 1950s, family doctors had been providing femininity certificates for female athletes since at least the 1940s. What changed at mid-century was that this process was taken out of the hands of national doctors, whose integrity was subject to suspicion, and given over to an apparently 'neutral' panel of scientists. Inherent in this is a desire to 'scientise' the process, as if by rendering it scientific it would become objective – and therefore fair.[35] The irony here is that the IOC (and others) turned to 'scientific' genetic and chromosomal tests for sex despite the fact that these are probably the most inappropriate of all testing regimes to successfully identify sex-linked physiological advantages in sport.[36]

Similar stories are told elsewhere about drug testing, where the desire to use the 'latest' scientific practices were disadvantaged by a thin or ambiguous conceptual base on which to decide *which* drugs should be banned or tested for in the first place (or, indeed, if dope should be banned at all).[37] Whatever objectivity could be claimed by the introduction of biomedical testing for both dope and gender in the 1960s, it was still the case that the desire to test – the assumption about 'normality' upon which testing was based – was essentially a social construction. What did not change from the 1930s to the 1960s was, for example, the cultural tension in many nations between femininity and competitive, aggressive sport. After all, other genotypes also provide helpful physiological features; Marfan Syndrome produces tall, slender bodies with clear advantages in some sports, epitomised by American volleyball player Flo Hyman (who died in 1986 at the age of 34 as a result of her condition); XYY athletes can be more aggressive and active than other phenotypical males; many studies have shown that height – which is significantly affected by genetic make-up – is a major component of athletic success.[38] Asking provocative questions about why we consider some metrics important in regulating athletic bodies, and ignore others entirely, would be a useful avenue for further research.

British doctors, scientists and administrators certainly played a role in the introduction of drug and gender testing. The IOC formed a proto-medical committee in the early 1960s to deal with dope and gender testing, which was formalised as a more general Medical Committee in 1967 (eight years after the BOA formed a medical committee); it was headed until 1966 by Sir Arthur Porritt (Box 5).[39] Shortly after the IOC introduced genetic screening for female athletes BAS(E)M arranged for a 'sex test kit' to be made available to sports governing bodies – presumably to enable them to avoid any possible embarrassments by testing athletes before they travelled to international events.[40]

Doping was also a topic discussed in some of the first BAS(E)M seminars in the late 1950s, and in 1964 the organisation drew up a draft policy on drugs, including what should and should not be banned.[41] It was a British scientist who introduced the first tests for amphetamine, although these were not initially designed for the purposes of sport. Professor Arnold Beckett had been working on 'drug distribution and metabolism and elimination in man' at Chelsea College, University of London, since 1958, but was encouraged in 1965 by a colleague at a conference to consider offering his expertise – particularly his methods of rapidly detecting traces of amphetamine in body fluids – to sporting organisations.[42] These tests were trialled for the first time in the UK, in 1965, at the cycling competition, the Tour de Britain ('Milk Race') and at the 1966 Football World Cup (for the purposes of experimentation rather than elimination). The straightforward accounts given of the development of this testing by Beckett in retrospective pieces is somewhat undermined by the recollections of Professor Harry Thomason, a student at the time:

> I was doing my PhD on hearts, and I wanted to look at people in a long endurance event . . . And they said well why don't you go on the Tour of Britain . . . it was announced a week before I went that I was going to do drug testing, in the press. I knew nothing about it. My own university refused to help me, but a man called Arnold Beckett from King's College London said he would help me, and we started drug testing under the Institute of Sports Medicine auspices.[43]

It is interesting to see the Institute mentioned in that account; of all the organisations involved with British sports medicine at mid-century it is the most archivally elusive, and seems to have contributed relatively little to sports medicine compared to the Sports Council, BAS(E)M or the

BOA. The Institute of Sports Medicine was founded in 1963 by BAS(E)M, the BOA and the Physical Education Association, who (despite their own scarce resources) raised several thousand pounds to put towards its overheads and first projects.[44] It was intended to represent the academic side of British sports medicine (or as it describes itself, 'a body of high academic standing'), while BAS(E)M was to be a membership organisation.[45] Membership of the Institute was by nomination rather than by application, which could be interpreted as a reaction against the full opening of BAS(E)M membership in 1961. It 'exist[ed] mainly to raise funds for research and education in sports medicine generally [and] its affairs [were] run by an Academic Board'.[46]

What the story of Professor Beckett and his Institute-backed amphetamine testing does make clear, however, is that the increased interest in and funding for sports medicine was beginning to attract the attention of researchers who might not otherwise have become involved with athletes. This gave organisations like BAS(E)M a new role – that of intermediaries. BAS(E)M in particular tried to configure itself as an intermediary between the world of sport, and of 'elite' scientific research, a process best illustrated by the Mexican Research Project into the effects of altitude, discussed below.[47]

Several members of the new sports medicine organisations were only peripherally involved in sports medicine practice (particularly treatment), or changes in the direction and scope of sports medicine, although almost all had some role to play in defining and policing athletic bodies. What was being created was a network of professionals in sport, science and medicine, at the core of which was a relatively select group (numbering perhaps two or three dozen) of sports medicine practitioners of the Hill and Abrahams type. These were those men who had a personal interest in sport and a professional interest in medicine (and they were still overwhelmingly male). Yet among these enthusiasts there were now those who regarded or engaged with sports medicine as a clear career choice.[48] Likewise, there could now be researchers who came to sports medicine not through personal interest, but rather because sports offered access to a range of human guinea pigs, available funding and specialist research centres.[49] Indeed, some athletes and their representatives felt the need in the 1960s to emphasise to this burgeoning group of researchers that athletes ought not to be unnecessarily experimented on, or have their training regimes disrupted by laboratory testing.[50]

In 1967 a review by the Sports Council identified three 'types' of sports medicine specialists; '[s]urgeons . . . perhaps with specialisms in orthopaedics or accident surgery', '[m]edical specialists, perhaps with the Diploma in Physical Medicine and Rehabilitation', or general practitioners (GPs) with 'no specialist knowledge or skills except those obtained by interest in and close association with their sport'.[51] (Of course, this list ignores physiologists, sports scientists and all those professions allied to medicine). This diversity of practitioners was matched by a diversity of sites, from the specialist laboratory through the temporary athlete's clinic to first-aid on the running track. The treatment aspect of sports medicine was increasingly being regularised and standardised, while enhancement and policing were gaining importance, funding, and attention at the international as well as the national level.

### The Olympics and international sports medicine

The 1956 Games were the first that were held outside the northern hemisphere – in Melbourne, Australia. One novel feature of international sport at the mid-century is a new concern about the environmental conditions at sporting venues – the jet-lag of attendance at Melbourne in 1956, heat in Rome in 1960, and altitude in Mexico City in 1968. First aid, a more long-standing concern, was to be provided by St John Ambulance in Melbourne, but other medical provision was apparently hampered by a national shortage of nurses and orderlies; as a consequence heavy use was made of medical personnel from the Australian Army and Royal Australian Air Force.[52] Otherwise medical man- (and woman-) power and equipment came from the Red Cross, donations from private companies, and voluntary work from individuals – some (twelve) of the latter being recruited from an advert in the *Medical Journal of Australia*.[53]

A 'Medical Centre' rather than a hospital was built in the Olympic Village, as the Medical Committee decided to 'provide treatment for minor or short-term ailments [only]. Any serious cases were to be evacuated to a civil hospital'.[54] Despite this the so-called Medical Centre was almost as well equipped as any previous Olympic Village hospital, with 24 beds, x-ray equipment, physiotherapy, chiropody and a separate dental centre. Visiting teams brought around six dozen doctors with them, supplemented and supported by further Australian doctors in the village and at event sites, alongside the usual emergency medical staff, first-aid facilities, ambulances, etc. Los Angeles had set a trend for public health, as the medical sub-committee was required to 'ensure that all possible hygienic steps were taken to maintain the health of residents', and there were '[t]wo senior Health Inspectors [who] kept kitchen cleanliness and sanitary arrangement under continuous review'.[55] 1663 athletes were treated, and 119 were sent to local hospitals.[56]

The increase in medical provision overseas was mirrored in services at home. From at least 1928 the BOA had provided general information to team members via a Team Handbook. The first editions had limited medical advice; in 1928 the handbook merely mentioned that there was a team doctor who should be consulted in case of illness or injury; in 1936, '48 and '52 the advice given was a variant on the following:

> A complete Medical service will be provided by the XVth Organising Committee. If any Competitor should require to see the Honorary Medical Officer he should immediately inform his Team Manager.[57]

In the 1956 Team Handbook this advice is increased, in particular in reference to 'public health' or hygiene issues and problems relating to the long-haul travel. Competitors were warned over several pages about dysentery, told to take malarial preventatives (the touch-downs were in 'known malarious areas'), to take four or five days to 'adjust' to the Australian climate, and advised on how to cope with heat and avoid sunburn and athlete's foot.[58]

A desire to define the athletic body was reasserted at Rome in 1960, where the Medical Scientific Committee introduced not only the expected comprehensive medical services (a large Dispensary-cum-hospital in the Village, and 37 first-aid posts, etc.) but also a card-record system. Though medical cards had long been used for injury reporting, the Rome scheme was specifically designed to include physiological and anthropological material, and was divided into eight sections, 'personal, genealogical, general, anmestic sports, clinical, anthropometric, bio-chemical, anmestic sports [and] psycho-physiological'.[59] Such investigation was almost certainly driven by the fact that Italy had a strong and well established 'Federation of Sports Medicine Doctors', including Giuseppe La Cava, who was involved in the introduction of the Olympic Medical Archive scheme (see Box 7).[60]

Of the 253 doctors available to athletes and the public at the Rome Olympiad, 172 were affiliated to FIMS, while 62 came from the armed forces and 19 from voluntary services such as the Red Cross. They were supported by 160 nurses and masseurs, 30 physiotherapists, and 208 stretcher-bearers. The Dispensary (in reality more like a hospital) offered special treatment in dentistry, otology, gynaecology, and orthopaedics as well as surgical, radiological and physiological facilities. The equipment list adds a helicopter and several vehicles to the usual material goods of first-aid kits, UV lamps, etc. The interest in public health continued; 554 checks were made on 'persons suspected of having contagious diseases'; a 'campaign against flies, mosquitoes, and other harmful insects' was waged with 'new modern pulverisation and spray equipment'; finally, a system of 'hygiene surveillance and control' was introduced for 'foodstuffs, beverages, and . . . temporary lodging[s]'.[61] Nearly 3000 people were treated, although this figure includes the public, accompanying personnel, and journalists as well as the athletes themselves.

The British Olympic Handbook carried more advice on health in 1960 (although from a twenty-first century standpoint the fact that the handbook was sponsored by Rothman's Pall Mall cigarettes may seem ironic). Two pages of advice covered the climate, training regimes, sleeping conditions, diet, the dangers of sunshine, and who to turn to for medical help. 1960 was also the first year when the BOA took out insurance for the team; a Personal Accident Insurance cover of up to £1000 for both athletes and officials – although notably this cover did *not* include 'sports accidents incurred in training or competition'.[62]

The services at the 1964 Tokyo Olympics were again based around a central Village Hospital, by now a necessary feature of Olympic medical provision. The Medical and Hygienic Committee was set up in May 1960 and was 'made up of members of sanitation authorities of the Ministry of Health and Welfare' local government administration officers, and 'others concerned including sports physicians of university hospitals'.[63] Alongside the hospital, emergency 'Village Clinics' were set up in the various 'detached villages' and other Olympic sites. The report claims that over 9000 medical staff were involved with the games (4600 nurses, 1900 doctors, and 2600 auxiliary staff); these numbers are apparently inflated by the inclusion of all the staff at the contracted hospitals which promised to provide emergency beds if necessary.[64]

Sanitation was a key concern; food vendors in streets near the sites and villages were inspected as well as the official caterers. There were a few scares at the games, including a swarm of flying ants, a case of cholera in Tokyo, and one mass-poisoning of a scout troop ('[f]ortunately, food intended for the athletes and officials was not involved').[65] Over 3000 athletes received treatment for orthopaedic or first-aid emergencies, and more than 4500 people received treatment for internal injuries (though this figure may include some members of the public). The organisers in Tokyo claimed that the increased use of their facilities was a consequence 'of the superior facilities and medical advice available'.[66] They also claimed that a significant number of the injuries they treated were a consequence of previous injuries, or damage done during training rather than competition, suggesting that many athletes were getting more limited treatment at home.

It is the case that for British athletes, at least, the intense medical supervision at the Olympics was sometimes an exception rather than the rule. Outside the Olympics few British athletes had contact with these Olympic medical officers or the BOA (access to sports doctors and other medical professionals depended rather on the specific sport).[67] Even the research done by interested organisations like the BOA did not always translate quickly into practice; in fact the sports medicine research which surrounded the Mexican Olympiad was one of the first examples of extensive research which was subsequently practically applied (and which took place outside the Olympic year). Some in sports medicine, Roger Bannister in particular, complained that studies of the late 1950s and 1960s had not been translated from sports medicine theory to sports medicine practice.[68]

In Mexico in 1968 the medical services were overseen by the Ministry of Health and Public Welfare – again integrating specific medical care, preventative treatment, and general sanitary and hygienic activity. Nine hundred and thrity-two medical personnel attended the medical centres/minature hospitals at the Olympic Villages and the many first-aid tents and rooms at each Olympic site; 1867 athletes were treated (and 837 non-competing team members).[69] The Official Report of the Mexican Olympics is one of the least forthcoming about the medical provision for athletes – an unwillingness to highlight the injuries encountered and treatment given may have been a reflection of the controversy surrounding the health risks of altitude (see below).

Generally, however, provision by the end of the 1960s was largely formalised – Rule 37 of the IOC's charter dictated the requirement for an Olympic Village and other rules and regulations had been introduced over the 1950s and 1960s laying down minimum requirements for the care of visiting athletes and spectators. By the time dope and gender tests were codified into the IOC's participation rules the framework for Olympic medical services was mostly standardised; large treatment centres, including minor surgery, at all major residential sites; first aid, including physiotherapy, at all sites of competition; medical coverage and supervision of events such as the marathon, and boxing. All host committees now sought to involve some systematic scientific research, or at least facilities for such, into the medical and hygienic programme. Mexico had a 'temporary . . . laboratory for human biological and genetic research'.[70] Presumably it was this laboratory which undertook the newly introduced femininity tests, although the subject of gender testing is not mentioned in the Official Report. This is strange, given that one of the IOC's lead experts in gender testing was Dr Eduardo Hay, a professor of gynaecology and obstetrics at the Faculty of Medicine, University of Mexico.[71]

There are some parallels in the development of services at the Olympic Games and in the UK. As mentioned above, the advice given directly to British competitors increased significantly. Likewise, research facilities were built, surveys undertaken, and grants and awards for sports medicine research were instituted. Increasingly, home nations as well as host nations developed schemes for training, screening, health checks, dietary advice, acclimatisation and so on in the years between Olympics. These were still aimed firmly at the elite athlete, a situation which was not to change until after 1970. Most significantly, of course, athletes were asked first to contribute to a medical definition of the athletic body through the dozens of physiological studies and tests; and secondly to submit themselves to biomedical testing which could result in disqualification if their bodies did not measure up.

## New organisations, new rules, new bodies

These new athletic bodies were subject to new rules, many of which were outlined and then enforced by the proliferating sports medicine organisations of the 1950s and 1960s. First was BAS(E)M, and a brief account of its founding was given in the last chapter. By the first AGM in February 1953 the ambitions of the organisation were clear, as Abrahams told the meeting that 'the Association had been founded with the aim of making it the authoritative body on every medical aspect of athletics and exercise'.[72] Abrahams gave three examples of the sort of work he envisaged BAS(E)M doing – investigating the effect of violent exercise during polio incubation, the possible dangers of boxing, and the effect of exercise upon girls and women. 'Research would play an important part in the Association's activities' involving biopsies of muscles, investigations of 'negro sprinters', exploring anthropometry and atavism, and engaging in studies of the biology on fatigue.[73]

In fact BAS(E)M's contribution to active research into the nature of the athletic body was minimal in the early years. In the 1960s its main organisational activity consisted of lectures and seminars, as it did not have the funds available to arrange research programmes or even large-scale conferences. For example: BAS(E)M was approached in 1954 by the National Association of Organisers and Lecturers in Physical Education, who wanted advice on the possible negative medical sequelae of schoolboy boxing. BAS(E)M met with the Amateur Boxing Association and then 'dr[ew] up a questionnaire on the subject' which, rather than circulating or managing themselves, they sent 'to the Medical Research Committee to enlist their help'.[74]

What BAS(E)M could do, and did effectively, was forge links with other organisations who *did* have money or influence; notably the BOA, the MRC, and later the Sports Council. Most significant sports medicine projects between 1953 and 1970 were the consequence of co-operation between several organisations and institutions. This is despite the fact that most of these organisations were also often in conflict for priority, prestige, and power over the athletic body.

BAS(E)M was fairly small and homogenous in its early years, because only medically qualified people could be full members, with 'scientists' accepted as 'honorary' or 'associate' members. By 1956 it had a membership of just 106 people.[75] In that year the Research Board for the Correlation of Medical Science and Physical Education closed down; this organisation had been formed in 1942 to address war-time concerns about population fitness and school sport. It was associated with the remedial gymnastics movement and counted many physiotherapists as members. In direct response to the disappearance of this organisation BAS(E)M opened its membership to physiotherapists in 1958, recognising that those interested in sports now had no appropriate organisation to join (they were allowed to become Associates, like the scientists).[76] This was followed in 1961 by the full opening of membership to anyone with a professional qualification in medicine or health care, or a professional interest in sport; membership doubled between 1961 and 1963 (from around 100 to well over 200; by 1968 it was over 450).[77]

In the 1960s BAS(E)M sought to broaden membership participation by introducing 'provincial meetings' – at first these consisted only of one conference a year, held at Loughborough.[78] The topic for the first provincial meeting in 1961 was, tellingly, 'Are Athletes Different?', and the overwhelming majority of the papers presented suggested that they were. The only notable exception to the rule that BAS(E)M concentrated on the elite, national-level was one provincial meeting in the mid-1960s, held jointly with the Physical Education Association and Medical Officers of Health Association which considered 'Sport and the School Child'.

Otherwise, the activity of BAS(E)M is typified by the provision of expert advice relating to a very specific patient body. A good example is the approach by Kenneth 'Sandy' Duncan (1912–2005) on behalf of the BOA in 1955, asking BAS(E)M to offer an opinion on whether jet lag and environmental change might affect women's menstrual cycles, and therefore their performance at the Melbourne Olympics in 1956. A sub-committee 'to consider the problems of Women Athletes' was formed, and concluded that no particular problems should arise.[79] In October 1955, BAS(E)M arranged for a 'panel of experts to answer similar questions on the treatment of injuries put to them by Olympics Games Coaches'.[80] In 1960 they gave advice on the possible environmental problems at the Rome Olympics, in 1964 they drew up their advice on doping, in 1965 they published a booklet on the *Medical Aspects of Boxing* (the proceedings of a conference held two years earlier) and in 1968 they held a special meeting to discuss the issue of altitude, prompted by the Mexico City Games.

Attempts to relocate the athletic body from the elite sphere into the community were actively unsuccessful. Between 1957 and 1958 BAS(E)M tried to provide a clinic for sports injuries at the Middlesex Hospital. Middlesex had been the site of the first clinic for athletes in the UK, initially run by Ben Woodard and varying in success and extent according to the registrar running it after he retired in 1953.[81] In 1957 representatives of BAS(E)M asked the resident orthopaedic surgeon, Mr Philip Wiles (a BAS(E)M member) to organise 'Saturday Evening Clinics' to run from 5–8pm. These were to be open to any sports injury, so long as 'the person [had been] injured on that day' and that they had 'a note from [their] Secretary or Captain'.[82]

Sports Injuries Clinics will be a key topic for the next chapter, but after 1970 these were explicitly facilities for the lay or 'normal' body. BAS(E)M's clinic is subtly different – for one thing, it required letters from team secretaries and captains, a level of formality ruling out many amateur sportsmen or casual sports injuries. For another, BAS(E)M specifically contacted elite and even professional sports clubs to invite them to participate; invites went to the Marylebone Cricket Club, the Rugby Football Union, the Hockey Association, and even the (professional) Football Association. The latter 'advis[ed] their affiliated clubs of this new innovation'.[83] Although BAS(E)M also advertised in sports magazines to let amateur athletes know that the service was available, the clinic – originally intended as a pilot study whose scheme could 'roll out' to other hospitals – was closed in late 1958 due to low attendance.[84] Other calls for special injury clinics in the 1960s also tended to concentrate on the needs of the elite and performance athlete.[85]

As well as defining the athletic body, as both a patient group and a clinical object, BAS(E)M was also involved in defining the sports medicine expert. Although the broadening of the membership appears to show a step away from the traditional narrowing processes of specialisation/ professionalisation, these should be offset against other expressions of professional identity. For one thing there was the formation of the Institute of Sports Medicine in 1963, and for another there was the production of the first British journal dedicated to sports medicine. In the early 1960s 'special editions' of other journals did consider sports medicine; in 1963 arrangements were made for a special issue of the Physical Education Association's journal, *Physical Education*, and offers of possible 'special editions' also came from the medical journal *Practitioner*.[86] But in 1964 BAS(E)M began to publish the *Bulletin of the British Association of Sport and Medicine*, which changed its name in December 1968 to the *British Journal of Sports Medicine (BJSM)*. The shift in name mirrors a shift in content – as it evolved into the *Journal* it took more submitted papers (especially from overseas) rather than reproducing those given at various BAS(E)M seminars and conferences. The production of a journal is often considered to be a significant marker in the process of professionalisation, or of specialisation in medicine, which is discussed further in Chapter 6.

Many of BAS(E)M's most cordial professional relationships in the 1950s and 1960s were held with the BOA. Sometimes it is hard to establish where BAS(E)M ends and the BOA's own medical committees begin; in the 1950s the tendency was for the BOA to turn to BAS(E)M for advice on medical and training questions, often forming collaborative sub-committees. A slightly more independent committee was formed by the BOA in 1959 to consider the specific environmental problems of the Rome Olympics, although it was under the chairmanship of Porritt and drew members from BAS(E)M as well as the MRC and some governing bodies of sport. Technically this was an ad hoc committee, intended to reform and dissolve in tune with the quadrennial cycles of the Games themselves, but the awarding of the XIXth Games to Mexico City in 1963 provided the impetus to make the Medical Committee a permanent fixture.

*Sports medicine research*

The Mexican Research Project became the most expensive sports medicine research project undertaken by any British organisation before 1968, with a total expenditure of over £5000.[87] Significantly, the Project's purpose was to study the effect of altitude on athletic performance in order to protect athletes and improve their competitive chances; in other words, public money from the Sports Council and BOA was being used for sports medicine research, without any justifications relating to military strength or public health. The Project's aims were to investigate the 'altitude problem'; Mexico City sits at a height of 7500 feet (2286 metres) above sea level, and although only classified as mid-altitude this is still high enough to cause symptoms of altitude sickness, particularly in susceptible individuals. By the 1960s the winning margins of Olympic events were such that even a fall in performance of a few percent could easily make the difference between winning a medal and going home empty-handed.

The 'altitude problem' is discussed in much more detail elsewhere.[88] Altitude became a focal point for a range of conflicts, and caused a reconsideration in the UK of fundamental sports concepts like 'amateurism' by playing into highly politicised international debates. In the 1960s Olympic athletes were held to fairly rigorous rules regarding their amateur status, which limited the amount of 'special training' they were supposed to undertake. Athletes' representatives claimed that 'there will be those who would die' if they competed at altitude without adequate acclimatisation, so significant pressure was applied to the IOC to solve this problem by changing the rules about training or changing the site of the Olympics.[89] Some commentators – notably Roger Bannister, a member of BAS(E)M and the Sports Council at this time – insisted that the altitude problem threatened the amateur ideal of the Olympics.[90] The argument ran that no countries would want to send their athletes unprepared to altitude and so success at the games would depend on the financial resources of a country, i.e. its ability to send athletes to expensive high-altitude training camps. It was 'little wonder' wrote Bannister, 'that Russia and America have not so far complained, but smaller countries look to us for a defence of the amateur'.[91]

Of course some 'smaller' (read: 'poorer') countries did rather well out of altitude: Kenya and Mexico have populations which live at altitude and both took nine medals in 1968 compared to one each in 1964. The suggestion was made, of course, that the Mexican Organizing Committee had deliberately chosen Mexico City in order to unfairly advantage their own athletes. Here we see the complications of the need to 'standardise' the athlete; why should the 'standard' environment of the Olympics reflect that of the sea-level temperate countries and not those at altitude or in the tropics? A sports reporter in the *Daily Mail* made precisely this point in 1966:

> 'I am sorry Mexico City is 7,500ft. above sea level. I also regret that it is cold in Iceland, hot in Malaya, high in Nepal, inflationary in France, communist in Russia, earth-quakey in Chile, oily in Iraq, sandy in Egypt, intolerant in Ireland, foggy in Britain, revolting in West Africa, Democratic in the United States, malarial in the Congo, humid in Jamaica, indeterminate in Mali and another day altogether in Fiji. So do we start a decent Olympic club whose membership permanently excludes all countries which have something wrong with them? ... The enduring virtue of sport is its acceptance the challenge of physical environment.[92]

The BOA's research started in June 1965 with the first meetings of the ad hoc committee, which solicited funds from the newly formed Sports Council. Dr LGCE Pugh (Box 8) of the MRC co-ordinated the research programme, while the BOA was represented by Dr Raymond Owen (d.1985). Two members of the Amateur Athletic Association, the honorary secretary Arthur Gold and the national coach John le Masurier, were co-opted into the project. Finally, six middle-distance athletes were chosen as the project's guinea pigs.[93] The athletes undertook standardised training in the UK, along with extensive physiological testing and time trials, before attempting to repeat their activity in Mexico City in November 1965.

Dr Pugh, Dr Owen and Mr le Masurier all produced individual reports, which were synthesised by the BOA Medical Committee, and then finally released as an official report by the executive committee of the BOA in early 1966.[94] All cited four weeks of acclimatisation as sufficient to prevent negative health outcomes from competition, which was, perhaps not coincidentally, the maximum amount of 'special training' allowed in one year by the IOC. All admitted that four weeks would not be sufficient to prevent some diminution of performance. Reactions to this conclusion were mixed – there were still those who argued that the altitude problem threatened the 'fairness' of the Games, while others suggested that the spirit of amateurism dictated that one ought to take part for the love of the game, not simply to gain medals and accolades.

It was important to the BOA that they used this opportunity to articulate their authority. Personality clashes between Dr Pugh and the rest of the research team had led to ill-feeling about leaks of information to the press, and journalists baited Dr Pugh into criticising the official report once it was published.[95] The BOA sought to be *the* authority on altitude for all Olympic competitors and governing bodies of sports. The need for central authority could even be justified on a scientific and biomedical basis; the BOA's Medical Committee highlighted the problem of psychosomatic altitude sickness:

> [t]here has been a vast amount of irresponsible and uninformed statements made about Mexico City, and if people go there without understanding the true facts they will be liable to experience just those symptoms they have been told to expect.[96]

The altitude problem, and its solution (which included training camps for Olympic 'possibles' in St Moritz, Switzerland) established the BOA's Medical Committee as a permanent and authoritative source of medical advice and guidance.

The Mexican Research Project was also co-sponsored by one of the newest bodies involved in sports medicine, the Sports Council. The Sports Council met for the first time on Thursday 18 February 1965, under the chairmanship of Denis Howell MP (1923–98).[97] A sub-committee, the Research and Statistics Committee (chaired by Roger Bannister until 1972) dealt with most of the sports-medicine-related activities of the Sports Council.[98] It is notable, though, that the decision to co-fund the Mexican Research Project was made at the very first meeting of the Sports Council – even before the Research Committee had been properly formed.[99]

For a body created from an investigation into 'community' sports, it is interesting how quickly the needs of elite athletes became the priority for *medical* research (if not elsewhere in the Council). As well as agreeing to fund the Mexican Research Project (to the tune of £2500), the Sports

Council also resolved to 'assist the development of work in exercise physiology' by 'recommending support by the Department of Education and Science for the training of . . . suitably qualified candidates'.[100] Indeed the Sports Council showed a keen interest in the academic and research side of sports medicine, and it was central to the founding of the first dedicated sports medicine research centre; by April 1966 the Council already had extensive plans for a 'permanent research centre' for sports medicine, with an annual budget in the region of £30,000.[101]

The MRC was approached initially for support and advice about setting up such a laboratory, and later offered formal grants, funding and loans of equipment and staff. A mobile (rather than permanent) centre was opened at Crystal Palace in 1967, as a pilot study. Staffed by one full time researcher (Mr CTM Davies) who was supported by the Environmental Physiology Research Unit at the London School of Hygiene and Tropical Medicine the laboratory proved popular with researchers, being booked out six months in advance until well into the 1970s. Once this small laboratory – fitted out with 'standard' physiological research equipment – had been opened, BAS(E)M and the Institute of Sports Medicine were approached to gauge their interest in a more permanent facility.[102] Representatively, BAS(E)M was most interested in the availability of conference and lecture facilities; the Institute in the research facilities.[103] The Greater London Council (GLC) was also involved in the venture – the GLC's architects drew up plans for a permanent research facility of around 600 square feet which was opened in the late 1970s; it was organised in close association with several higher education colleges in London, to secure students not just as researchers, but also as vital guinea pigs.[104]

### British sports medicine: elite bodies only?

The Sports Council was not just interested in research and laboratory studies. It also showed a keen interest in sports medicine as a clinical practice. In 1967 it produced a special report (written by the deputy director of the Research and Statistics Committee, Mr DD Molyneux) on the treatment of sports injuries in Britain.[105] This 1967 report – *Sports Injuries, a General Background to the Position in Britain* – gives three specific reasons why 'sports injuries can justify separate consideration from other injuries'.[106] Firstly 'most individuals who sustain injury . . . [in this way] . . . are keen to return to their sport as quickly as possible'.[107] This assertion, along with a similar argument that athletes needed to be restored to health as quickly as possible is a deeply problematic argument; the suggestion is that non-athletes are ambivalent about becoming fit and healthy again, or about regaining mobility!

Secondly, Molyneux argued that the injuries sustained in taking part in sport needed particularly early intervention and integrated treatment between doctors, coaches and physiotherapists. This argument is somewhat more grounded in the practical specificities of sport – but again, the counter-suggestion that everyone else can put up with non-immediate intervention, treatment delay, and poorly co-ordinated care is nonsensical. Finally, the report makes a specific case for sports injuries: it describes some of them as discrete clinical entities which deserved discrete clinical study and treatment. In a particularly reflexive argument the report uses the emergence of sports medicine organisations (BAS(E)M and the Institute), and publications (such as the *Bulletin of the British Association of Sport and Medicine* and Williams' *Sports Medicine*) as evidence that sports medicine was already a 'ghost' specialty, which required a distinctive form of medical intervention.

In the following month (September 1967) the Sports Council resolved 'that inquiries should be made with the Ministry of Health to ascertain in what circumstances clinics for sports injuries might operate whether at hospitals or rehabilitation centres'.[108] George Godber (1908–2009) the government's Chief Medical Officer, was approached by Bannister and '[d]iscussion followed on the possible steps which might be taken to gather evidence of user need for better and more co-ordinated services' particularly sports injuries clinics.[109] A protracted round of consultations, with BAS(E)M, the Institute, the British Orthopaedic Association and the British Association of Physical Medicine was instigated; eventually a grant of around £1000 was given in 1969 to Professor RC Browne at Newcastle to survey sports injuries as a 'pilot study'.[110] This funding was renewed in 1971 and 1972, and the conclusions of the survey – showing significant numbers of sports injuries among the general population, which appeared to receive inadequate treatment – led to the Sports Council's Sports Injuries Clinics scheme, which is discussed in the next chapter.

What is particularly significant about the sports injuries report and its consequences is that *at no point* was the 'special' nature of either the athlete or his/her injury questioned. In the case of the elite performer the athlete was a unique clinical entity; in the case of the mass of amateur sports men and women sports injuries required (at least according to the Sports Council) some form of special intervention. Despite this, the Council did not (yet) see sports medicine as a distinct clinical specialty, and in 1969 explicitly stated that: '[w]e do not share the view that 'sports medicine' can be regarded as sufficiently important to warrant treatment as a major specialty, e.g. by the development of national training programmes'.[111]

This negativity towards medical specialism can be partly attributed to the fact that this standpoint was drawn out of the Sports Council by the publication, in 1967, of the Council of Europe's report on the *Medical Aspects of Sport*.[112] This was the product of a working party of the European Public Health Committee, which had no British representatives.[113] The Sports Council was responsible for drawing up the official British response to the Council of Europe's report; this response is extraordinarily dismissive. It argued that *Medical Aspects of Sport* entirely failed to take into account the special nature of British healthcare provision and the differences between education systems across Europe. The Sports Council also criticised the medical and scientific assertions of *Medical Aspects of Sport*, and argued that its ideological basis was entirely alien to British sentiments about sport and health care.

*Medical Aspects of Sport* seemed to epitomise what British sports medicine was *not*. Its conclusions were particularly concerned with issues of policing which were not as significant in British sports medicine practice. In particular, the report discusses in great detail the screening of schoolchildren and makes strong links between sports medicine, physical education and school sports. Its model of public health is highly interventionist, recommending near universal health screening for all participants in all sports, possibly with doctors deciding what sort of exercise regimes specific individuals should follow. Arising from this is the recommendation that governments recognise sports medicine as a specialty and establish sports medicine centres for training and treatment. The total rejection of this report in the UK was not limited to representatives of elite sports and medical organisations, but also those working in school and leisure sports; according to the British Senior Inspector of Physical Education the report was 'misleading, misguided and inaccurate', and ought to be totally disregarded.[114]

Through the rejection of the interventionalist ideology of *Medical Aspects of Sports* the Sports Council articulated an idealised assertion of independence and individual autonomy in lifestyle. But this also extended to the regulation of professional activities, hence the dismissal of the idea that sports medicine should become a specialty; to the specific recommendation that the government recognise sports medicine, the Sports Council responds:

> This implies a more direct involvement of the government in the life of the citizen than is normally acceptable in Great Britain ... In the United Kingdom it is generally left to the professional bodies concerned with the medical education to advise which specialities should be recognised.[115]

So there are two main reasons why the report proved so challenging. First was the high level of policing activity promoted, including mass screening of most of the population before they could participate in sport. Secondly, and more significantly, the report discusses school sports and casual exercise alongside elite sports. Most of the Council of Europe's recommendations centred on the schoolchild, the amateur sportsman and the casual athlete. As we have already seen, in Britain, sports medicine had turned away from these issues to focus instead on the elite athlete, who, as a different sort of clinical being, had very different needs to the general population.

By the mid-twentieth century British sports medicine had a distinct 'flavour'. Ironically, for a nation which figured its idealised sportsmen as amateurs who participated in sport as a leisure activity or as a hobby, it appeared to have constructed its sports doctors as elite, professional specialists. Although they may still have offered their services voluntarily, they were there for the treatment and enhancement of the national or international-level athlete, of the healthy competitive sportsman or woman. They did not, by-and-large, treat children, or the 'general public', or worry about national fitness and physical exercise.[116] So while the Council of Europe suggested that British sports medicine was negligent in these areas, the Sports Council responded by arguing that such activity was the true remit of the family doctor, general practitioner or school medical officer; specialists in sports medicine worked elsewhere.

The Sports Council (and others) also quibbled with the intellectual and scientific basis of the Report which, as the Senior Inspector of Physical Education to the London County Council wrote, 'assumes that there is a medical "deposit of the truth" on all sports matters'.[117] We have already seen how British sports medicine was drawing boundaries around the athletic body, and in the process surveying, examining and experimenting on it; this was an active and ongoing process – and most of the institutions of sports medicine justified their existence in part through their ability to fund and co-ordinate this work. Obviously the representatives of British sports medicine did not agree with the suggestion that these boundaries had been clearly drawn and were already thoroughly understood.

### Influence and authority

The quote above about the 'deposit of truth', refers specifically to boxing, and the controversy about boxing demonstrates one final point about the Sports Council and its activity, and will be the final aspect of their work that we consider before turning to the Institute of Sports Medicine. The boxing inquiry in the late 1960s proved difficult to organise, and highlights one of the natural advantages the BOA and the Sports Council had over BAS(E)M in terms of their authority over sports organisations. The Sports Council obviously had financial incentives to offer to sports bodies, the BOA could do the same to a limited extent, and also had some administrative control over Olympic participation. BAS(E)M did not have clear access to either of these sources of enforcement or authority, and as a consequence it was sometimes the BOA or the Sports Council which was approached when a medical intervention was needed, as was the case for the boxing inquiry.

Some of the history of the relationship between medical authority and boxing is discussed elsewhere; the story is far from clear cut, with doctors both condemning and warmly supporting the practice of boxing through-out the twentieth century.[118] Supporters of boxing complicated the picture by introducing the notion that there was good and bad boxing, and that there were appropriate and inappropriate boxing bodies; these defini-tions were not applied universally. Thus professional boxing – with more bouts and its inherent 'moral' inferiority due to being a financial as well as a 'sporting' encounter – could be worse than the noble art of amateur boxing.[119] On the other hand, well regulated professional boxing might distinguish itself from unregulated illegal boxing for money, or from poorly regulated and casually supervised amateur boxing.[120] Boxing for children might be decried while boxing for young army recruits was an essential formative for body and character, etc.

In the late 1960s a proposed enquiry by the Royal College of Physicians into the after-histories of boxers had been scuppered by the British Boxing Board of Control, who 'did not feel they could permit a research worker to interview boxers, whose case histories were confidential'.[121] The Sports Council offered to intervene – to act as a go-between for the institutions of medicine and sport. Less than four months later agreement between the two parties had been secured, and the 'Boxing Inquiry' took place, on con-dition that 'the BBBC should be shown any reports before publication'.[122] The Sports Council also gave financial sponsorship costing in total £2617, about equivalent to their contribution to the Mexican Research Project.[123]

The aim in 1968 was to expand this project to include amateur as well as professional boxing, but the final report – issued by the Royal College of Physicians in 1969 – only considered professional boxing in any detail.[124] This was apparently due to the absence of systematic records for most amateur boxers. So when the Amateur Boxing Association met with the Sports Council to discuss the inquiry in 1970, amateur boxing's medical supporters had a ready-made defence: professional and amateur boxing were different sports and should not be compared, and since there was no evidence from amateur boxing, no conclusions about the dangers of amateur boxing could be drawn. In any case, they argued, the sporting life of a professional boxer now was so different to that of the previous genera-tion that no useful predictions could be drawn from these statistics about the ill-effects of 'modern' boxing in the 1960s or 1970s.[125] The Amateur

Boxing Association was persuaded, however, to make a commitment to keeping more statistically useful records, and to 'welcome and co-operate with any further research directed at amateur boxing'.[126] In return the Sports Council's Research Committee recommended that:

> sympathetic consideration should be given to an application from the Amateur Boxing Association for grant towards the additional administrative costs of keeping detailed records of amateur boxers' careers throughout the country.[127]

The Sports Council therefore had considerable resources with which to assert or buy authority in sports medicine – at least compared with the other sports medicine groups considered here. In its first five years of activity (1965/6 to 1970/1) the Research Committee paid out nearly £35,000 in sports medicine or sports science grants (representing about 20% of the total grant spending of the whole Council).[128] The expenditure of the Sports Council gives mathematical support for my assertion that sports medicine in Britain focused on the elite, not the lay, athlete. Up until 1970 over 90% of the Sports Council's Research Committee money went on either elite sport or basic physiological research, rather than studies of fitness, physical education or the 'lay' body; the only exceptions to the concentration on the elite or physiology was a £200 expenditure on a project on the capacity for exercise in young children and the eventual expenditure of £2289 on the Sports Injuries survey at Newcastle (more than half of this was spent *after* 1970 with Browne's two extensions).[129] This pattern changed dramatically in the early 1970s with a £5715 project on the effect of exercise on 'normal' (and post-coronary) middle-aged men; as such it is a clear indicator of the changes to come.

Without these sources of influence, BAS(E)M and the Institute of Sports Medicine had to rely on their professional expertise, and their connections with governing bodies of sport and other organisations. The Institute certainly had grand intentions, laid out in its six objectives; the first three concentrated on research – 'to promote the scientific study of fitness and the treatment of sports injuries', to encourage other groups to engage in relevant research, and provide equipment, staff and accommodation for such research.[130] Two 'objects' related to pedagogy and training – the desire to 'conduct courses of instruction' and to establish a library. Finally the Institute asserted its right to co-operate with whomsoever they pleased to fulfil the first five objects. How well the Institute achieved these aims is difficult to establish; in 1968 contemporaries remarked that it was 'quite commendable' but had achieved little.[131] As well as the drug research mentioned previously, in 1966 and 1967 it successfully ran courses in exercise physiology and sports medicine at Loughborough's Summer School, and in 1969 co-organised a meeting with the Occupational Medicine and Orthopaedics sub-sections of the Royal Society of Medicine.[132]

What the Institute desired to do overlapped significantly with the Sports Council and BAS(E)M's activities; '[a]mongst its objects [were] the establishment of a permanent research centre [and] the creation of clinics for the treatment of sports injuries'.[133] Neither of these emerged until after 1970. What did happen in the 1960s was a fairly spectacular falling out between BAS(E)M and the Institute, which has coloured the relationship between the two organisations until well into the twenty-first century. This situation was precipitated by the resignation of Porritt; he had been the chairman of the Institute as well as a central member of BAS(E)M, and resigned when he was appointed the Governor General of New Zealand in 1967. At a meeting on 10 April 1968 changes were made to the constitution of the Institute which dictated that BAS(E)M representative was to be *invited* by the Institute rather than *nominated* by BAS(E)M. Although this may seem a relatively minor assertion of independence, it was complicated by a further disenfranchisement of BAS(E)M members, who had not had notice of (and not been invited to) this April meeting. Legal advice solicited by BAS(E)M suggested that the Institute did not have the authority to alter its membership rules this way. Consequently BAS(E)M, represented by its chairman Dr GG Browning, made a direct, formal complaint to the new chairman of the Institute, Mr Norman Capener (1898–1975).[134]

Capener promised to discuss the problems at the next Institute meeting, but the tensions did not ease; Capener's written response inflamed the situation as a meeting of BAS(E)M declared it 'replete with inaccuracies' and claimed that 'Mr Capener's views as stated were in conflict with the [Institute's] registered constitution'.[135] BAS(E)M decided against pursuing legal action over 'unconstitutuional' activities by the Institute, but tried to establish a joint working party.[136] The situation did not resolve, although there was a feeling that 'for the good of sports medicine generally' the dispute should not be made public.[137] The Institute appointed a new chairman, Lord Luke (b.1933), in 1970, and he approached BAS(E)M to 'clear the air'.[138] But a private meeting concluded that he 'had not been told about the difficulties of the past few years'.[139] Despite these difficulties, Browning was nominated to act as a representative for BAS(E)M at the Institute, under the premise that failure to co-operate would 'look most peculiar' unless the public were informed of 'all the facts of relations between Association and Institute' which was a step declared still 'not to be in the best interests of sports medicine'.[140]

The relationship did not become close. While the activities of the Institute in the period considered here were relatively small and minor, consisting of a few training and education schemes and some public and private meetings and seminars, it did expose the fault lines and conflicts within the small world of British sports medicine. The existence of such conflicts – and BAS(E)M's clear desire to keep them away from the public, and even its full membership – is evidence of the formation of a professional identity in sports medicine. Through such small, and often deeply personal, negotiations the boundaries of authority in sports medicine were being drawn.

## Conclusion

This tense relationship between the Institute and BAS(E)M was not the only conflict within sports medicine; the Mexican Research Project was an extraordinarily fractious event, both in regard to the criticism of Mexico as a location and of the IOC, but also the media coverage of the BOA's activities, and the conflicts between Dr Pugh/the MRC and the BOA.[141] The Sports Council's records show similar tussles in international sports medicine. For example – letters between members of the Council in 1966 discuss the 'problem' of Ernst Jokl (1907–97), who approached the Sports Council in 1966 asking for money towards the founding of a headquarters for the International Committee for Sport and Physical Education (instrumental in the Sport for All scheme discussed in the next chapter).[142] Opinions on the value of his research, his standing in sports medicine, and his actual authority within the International Committee varied considerably; apparently he had made similar approaches to both the Spanish and US governments, 'without the knowledge of his research committee, even of its secretary' (his request was turned down).[143] Most conflicts of the 1960s can be characterised as jostling for territory, physical, financial, and intellectual, within sports medicine.

At the centre of this territory, of course, was a patient body – the athletic body. Athletes were clearly recognised as a discrete subpopulation; to return to the BOA for an example, when anti-diarrhoeal drugs were sourced for the British Olympic Team travelling to Rome it was not enough that they had been systematically scientifically tested on healthy men and women, the athlete had to be reassured that the effect of 'streptotriad' on exercise and athletes had been specifically considered.[144] And it was not just the athletic *body* which differed – athletes were being credited with a different psychology. The mind of the athlete had been characterised in a variety of ways, ranging from the perfect stoic gentleman to the hysterical, superstitious, professional athlete. Increasingly, the mental fragility and suggestibility of the elite athlete came to be a consideration in sport. The BOA's desire to control information about altitude was couched in terms of the 'psychosomatic' diseases of altitude. Likewise, the 'compliancy' of athletes, their tendency to hide or downplay injuries, unwillingness to rest, etc., were topics for consideration at sports medicine meetings and in the pages of the medical press.[145]

The athlete's body and athlete's mind were being constructed as 'special'; signs and symptoms which were pathological in the normal body – an enlarged heart, blood in the urine, delayed onset of menstruation – could all now be normal, physiological adaptations in the athlete. Yet at the same time there were no significant calls in Britain for sports medicine to be considered as a specialism. Indeed, in 1963 Porritt insisted that '[t]he BAS(E)M has always been strenuously opposed to any suggestion that it is aiming to introduce yet another new specialty into Medicine'; we have already seen the Sports Council espousing the same views.[146] Instead of formal specialty, what sports medicine practitioners pursued were specialist sites and specialist authority; clinics, conferences, journals, research, laboratories. So while the athletes need not be treated by a Doctor of Sports Medicine, or a Sports Medicine Consultant, they were to be treated by experienced generalists, or by a team of experts who were all members of a sports medicine association, and worked (ideally) in a sports medicine clinic.

But this understanding of sports medicine is difficult to maintain, and attempts at this time to define sports medicine often highlight internal tensions. At one of BAS(E)M's provincial conferences in Loughborough, in 1963, one member presented a paper titled 'What is Sports Medicine?':

> It is an important branch of preventive medicine, aimed at preserving full health and working efficiency. The study of the trained athlete should not only be an end in itself, but the means to understanding norms to which all should aspire. The trained athlete differs from the 'average' member of the population as regards his physiology and response to injury and illness as much as does a child or an old person.[147]

The athletic body is a norm to which we should all aspire; yet it is as different from us as the very old or very young. The athletic body is a special entity; yet sports medicine does not need to be a formal specialty. For the ideological purpose of sport the athlete must be something to which the normal person can aspire; yet according to sports medicine they are supernormal, or even abnormal.

British sports medicine had so internalised the fact that sport was a distinct activity and sportsmen/women a distinct clinical type, that it found itself, after 1970, in conflict with the rest of the medical and governmental world. Here, sport was just one among hundreds of risky or rewarding activities, and sportsmen and women just a small proportion of millions of needy patients. To continue as a distinct specialism sports medicine had to find a way to reintegrate the lay body and the elite athletic body; the next chapter discusses this process.

## Notes

1 A Abrahams, 'Medical Aspects of Athletics' *BMJ* 1 (1955), 1026.
2 Most relevant are the various subcommittees of the Physical Education Association, the CCPR and the Ergonomics Research Society. The latter 'formed an ad hoc group for the study of physiological and psychological problems in sport' in 1958, hosting a conference in 1959 on 'the physiological and psychological aspects of athletics' which was based on some observations of athletes at the 1958 Commonwealth Games. This committee became the 'Fitness and Training Section' in 1961, but was disbanded in the late 1960s. National Archives [hence: NA]. FD23/89. *Medical Research and Sport*. Proceedings of the Ergonomics Research Society meeting with the CCPR, 19 Jun. 1959; Memorandum on the incorporation of the *Ad Hoc* group, 17 Apr. 1961; letter JE Cotes to Dr Russell-Smith, 16 Jan. 1963.
3 Wolfenden Committee on Sport, *Sport and the Community* (London: CCPR, 1960–61), p. 1.
4 For example, the Polish sprinter Ewa Kłobukowska who failed the 'close-up visual inspection of the genitalia' followed by a genetic test at the 1967 European Cup (Athletics). Presenting as XXY instead of the 'normal' XX her records were stripped from her and she was banned from competing in women's events. She subsequently married and gave birth to a son; culturally and socially female, she was not considered a woman for sport. Anon, 'Girl Athlete To Have New Sex Tests' *Daily Mirror*, 20 Sep. 1967. For more general critiques see: M Genel and A Ljungvist, 'Gender verification of female athletes' *Lancet* 366(2005), s41; BD Dickinson *et al.*, 'Gender verification of female Olympic athletes' *Medicine and Science in Sports and Exercise* 34 (2002), 1539-42.
5 G La Cava, 'Sports Medicine' *Lancet* 276 (1960), 1144.
6 'It is natural to ask whether there are any fixed limits to athletic performance and physical endurance. History – including the climbing of Everest last year – suggest that there are not.' Anon, 'A Great Runner' *BMJ* 1 (1954), 1143.
7 British political attempts to present British sport (particularly British 'amateurism') as a third way between the state-sponsored gymnasts of the USSR and the hot-housed American college athletes are discussed elsewhere. P Beck, 'Britain and the Cold War's "Cultural Olympics": Responding to the Political Drive of Soviet Sport, 1945–58' *Contemporary British History* 19 (2005), 169-85.
8 Wolfenden Committee, *Sport and the Community*, p. 1.
9 Problems caused by the multiple definitions of 'amateurism' within national sports groups, and in international sports organisations, also loom large.
10 Wolfenden Committee, *Sport and the Community*, p. 106.

11 Ibid., pp. 14-15.

12 Ibid., p. 104.

13 Centre for Sports Science & History, Birmingham University: Archives of the Sports Council [hence: CSSH]. SC(RS)(66)8a. Preliminary Plans for a Permanent Research Centre for Sports Medicine – a paper by Dr Edholm, 15 Apr. 1966.

14 [NA] FD23/89. *Medical Research and sport.* Note from Dr Russell to Mr Mears, 28 Jan. 1963.

15 [NA] FD23/89. Memorandum attached to Note from Dr Russell to Mr Mears, 23 Jan. 1963.

16 'Editorial', *BJSM* 1 (1964), 42; Archives of the British Olympic Association [hence: BOA] 34.23 MED INJUR. *Materials on Sports Medicine.* Report of the Olympic Medical Archives, Tokyo 1964 (ed. Toshiro Azuma).

17 British Association of Sport and Exercise Medicine Archives. [hence: BAS(E)M]. *AGM.* 19 Mar. 1954; *Minutes of the Executive Committee.* 9 Jan. 1969.

18 Anon, 'Injuries and treatment' *Athletics Weekly* 14.48 (1960), 3.

19 JGP Williams, 'Injuries and treatment' *Athletics Weekly* 14.50 (1960), 7.

20 Loughborough Training College provided teacher training and gained a reputation in particular for teaching in physical education. The constituent parts of Loughborough College had broken into separate colleges in the early 1950s, and were then gradually reintegrated into Loughborough University after 1966; sport and exercise science soon became one of the specialist areas of the new university. LM Cantor & GF Matthews, *Loughborough: From College to University* (Loughborough: Loughborough University, 1977). See also the evidence of Professor Harry Thomason in Reynolds & Tansey, *The Development of Sports Medicine*, pp. 18-19.

21 JGP Williams, *Sports Medicine*, (London: Edward Arnold, 1962). Vii; this quote is also highlighted in I Waddington, 'The Development of Sports Medicine' *Sociology of Sport Journal* 13 (1996), 176–96. 179.

22 CB Heald, *Injuries and Sport: A General Guide for the Practitioner* (Oxford: Oxford University Press, 1931); JGP Williams, Sports Medicine.

23 Donald Featherstone's manual, aimed at coaches and trainers without any medical training, went through two editions in the period under consideration. DF Featherstone, *Sports Injuries Manual for Trainers, Coaches, etc.* (London: Nicholas Kaye, 1954) [subsequent edition 1957].

24 See for example this account of a collapse at an athletics county championships (heated correspondence on the issue of medical supervision followed). GEJ McMillan, 'Letters to the Editor: First Aid' *Athletics Weekly* 11.4 (1957), 4-5.

25 HB Lee, 'Letter to the Editor: Marathons' *Athletics Weekly* 9.33 (1955), 15 & 17. See also the ongoing debate two years later about the timing and control of marathons: *Athletics Weekly* 11.15 (1957), 4; 11.17 (1957), 4-5; 11.18 (1957), 19.

26 Featherstone, *Sports Injuries Manual*; WD Jarvis, *A Medical Handbook for Athletic and Football Club Trainers* (London: Faber and Faber, 1955);

KG Sheard, '"Brutal and Degrading": The Medical Profession and Boxing, 1838–1984' *International Journal of the History of Sport* 15 (1998), 74–102.

27 R Owen, 'Letters to the Editor: Medical Facilities' *Athletics Weekly* 11.7 (1957), 5-6. 5; Stanley Miles, 'Medical Criteria in the Selection of Athletes' *Proceedings of the Royal Society of Medicine* 62 (1969), 921-4.

28 On the suspicions about competitors from the Eastern Bloc, see: Dickenson *et al.*, 'Gender Verification'; LJ Elsas, RP Hayes, K Muralidharan, 'Gender Verification At The Centennial Olympic Games' *The Journal of the Medical Association of Georgia* 86 (1997), 50-4; T Todd, 'Anabolic Steroids and Sport' in J Berryman & R Park (eds), *Sport and Exercise Science: Essays in the History of Sports Medicine* (Chicago: University of Illinois Press, 1992), pp. 319–50; EA Ferris, 'Gender Verification Testing in Sport' *British Medical Bulletin* 48 (1992), 1–15 and of course J Hoberman, *Mortal Engines: The Science of Performance and the Dehumanization of Sport*, (New Jersey: Blackburn Press, 1992).

29 Elsas *et al.*, 'Gender Verification', 250.

30 The irony of this situation, given the later revelations about Walsh's ambiguous gender, has led some writers to link Walsh to the introduction of sex testing; many articles on this subject start with her and Hermann Ratjen (a German high-jumper who competed as a woman in 1936). Although of course an autopsy in 1980 could have no effect at all on the sex testing introduced in the 1960s, some articles seem to infer as much: 'In the 1932 Olympic games the 100-meter sprint champion was found to have testes during a 1980 autopsy after her accidental death.' Elsas *et al.*, 'Gender Verification', 50; See also D Langlais, 'The Road Not Taken: The Sex Secret That Really Didn't Matter' *Running Times*, Oct. 1988.

31 GP Moon, A New Dawn Rising; An Empirical and Social Study Concerning the Emergence and Development of English Women's Athletics until 1960, PhD, Roehampton Institute, 1997, pp. 293–4.

32 Anon, 'She's Now A Man' *Daily Mirror*, 29 May 1936; DF Wickets, 'Can Sex in Humans Be Changed' *Physical Culture*, Jan. 1937.

33 'Olympic Games' *Time*, 10 Aug. 1936; 'Change of Sex' *Time*, 24 Aug. 1936.

34 See just as an example S Lynch, 'When men were men . . . and so were the women' *Guardian*, 7 Aug. 2004.

35 For further critiques on drug and gender testing see: L Wackwitz, 'Verifying the Myth: Olympic Sex Testing and the Category 'Woman'' *Women's Studies International Forum* 26 (2003), 553–60; IE Ritchie, 'Sex tested, Gender verified: Controlling Female Sexuality in the Age of Containment' *Sports History Review* 34 (2003), 80–93; LR Davis & LC Delano, 'Fixing the Boundaries of Physical Gender: Side Effects of Anti-Drug Campaigns on Athletics' *Sociology of Sport Journal* 9 (1992), 1–19.

36 V Heggie, 'Men in Women's Sport', in M Atkinson (ed.) *Battleground: Sport* (Greenwood Press, 2008) Vol I, pp. 278–84; on science and the IOC see also A Wrynn, 'The Human Factor: Science, Medicine and the International Olympic Committee, 1900–70' *Sport in Society* 2 (2004), 211–31.

37  P Dimeo, A History of Drug Use in Sport, 1875–1976, Beyond Good and Evil (London: Routledge, 2007).

38  Contemporary doctors also made the connection between Marfans' and the ethics of sex testing: Ferris, 'Gender Verification', 693. On height, see T Khosla, 'Unfairness of Certain Events in the Olympic Games' *BMJ* 2 (1968), 111–13.

39  Wrynn, 'The Human Factor'; A De Merode, 'The Development, Objectives and Activities of the IOC Medical Commission' in A Drix, HG Knuttgen & K Tittel (eds) *The Olympic Book of Sports Medicine: Vol I of the Encyclopaedia of Sports Medicine* (Oxford: IOC+FIMS, 1988), pp. 3-6.

40  Archives of the British Association of Sport and Exercise Medicine [Hence: BAS(E)M] *Minutes of the Executive Committee*, 7 Mar. 1970.

41  Anon, 'Doping and the Use of Chemical Agents to Modify Human Performance in Sport' *BJSM* 1 (1964), 40-2.

42  AH Beckett, 'Misuse of Drugs in Sport' *BJSM* 12 (1979), 185-94.

43  See the evidence of Profesor Harry Thomason in LA Reynolds & EM Tansey (eds), *The Development of Sports Medicine in Twentieth-Century Britain: Wellcome Witness Seminar* (London: Wellcome, 2009), pp. 19-20.

44  Around £7000. [BAS(E)M] Miscellaneous Paper c. Dec 1963.

45  [CSSH] SC(RS)(67)26. Note of a meeting with representatives of the Institute of Sports Medicine, 30 Nov. 1967.

46  [CSSH] SC(RS)(66)17. 'Sports Injuries – A General Background to the Position in Britain', 25 Aug. 1967.

47  V Heggie '"Only the British Appear to be Making a Fuss": The Science of Success and the Myth of Amateurism at the Mexico Olympiad, 1968' *Sport In History* 28 (2008), 213–35.

48  For example, Drs Peter Sperryn and JGP Williams (see the following chapter)

49  Dr LGCE Pugh (Box 8) is an obvious example.

50  'Top class amateur athletes already have many demands made upon their time: they should not be asked to act as experimental subjects except in investigations for which they are indispensable'. [NA] FD23/89, *Medical Research and Sport*. JE Cotes, 'The Athlete as Research Subject', a paper given at an Ergonomics Research Society and CCPR joint meeting in 1959.

51  [CSSH] SC(RS)(66)17 'Sports Injuries – A General Background to the Position in Britain', 25 Aug. 1967.

52  Melbourne Olympic Committee, *The Official Report of the Organising Committee for the Games of the XVI Olympiad Melbourne 1956*, (Melbourne: Organising Committee of the Melbourne Olympiad, 1958).

53  Ibid., p. 188.

54  Ibid., p. 191.

55  Ibid., pp. 188, 190.

56  Ibid., p. 193. The single largest category of injury or disease is 'Accidental injury' (630), followed by 'Other specified and ill-defined diseases' (156), 'Boil, abscess, cellulites and other skin infections' (131) and the common cold (81).

57 [BOA] 13.1 BOA HDBK (1928–64). *Team Handbooks*. Official Handbook of the XVth Olympiad, Helsinki, 1952.

58 [BOA] 13.1 BOA HDBK (1928–64). *Team Handbooks*. Official Handbook of the XVIth Olympiad, Melbourne, 1956.

59 In this translation, 'amnestic' probably means mental or psychological, rather than strictly relating to amnesia.

60 HE Robson, 'Obituary: Professor La Cava' *BJSM* 23 (1989), 198.

61 Rome Organising Committee, *The Official Report of the Organising Committee for the Games of the XVII Olympiad Rome 1960, Vol I* (Rome: Organising Committee of the Rome Olympiad, 1960), p. 637.

62 [BOA] 13.1 BOA HDBK (1928–64). *Team Handbooks*. Official Handbook of the XVIIth Olympiad, Rome, 1960, p. 6.

63 Tokyo Organising Committee, *The Official Report of the Games of the XVIII Olympiad Tokyo 1964, Vol I* (Tokyo: Kyodo Printing Co. Ltd, 1964), p. 485.

64 Ibid., p. 492.

65 Ibid., pp. 493–4.

66 Ibid., p. 492.

67 See the evidence of Dr Malcolm Bottomley in Reynolds & Tansey, *The Development of Sports Medicine*, p. 43.

68 'Cotes, in collaboration with Dr Roger Bannister, concluded from their studies on the effect of environmental temperature upon performance, that athletes accustomed to a temperate climate are unlikely to do well in warm climates without a period of heat acclimatisation, yet the management of the British Team to the 1960 Olympic Games made no use of these findings.' [NA] FD23/89. *Medical Research and Sport*. Draft of a Letter to Dr Lush, n.d. *c.* Jan. 1963.

69 Mexico Organising Committee, *Official Report of the Organising Committee of the Games of the XIX Olympiad Mexico, 1968, Vol 2* (Mexico: The Organising Committee of the Games of the XIX Olympiad, 1968), p. 169.

70 Ibid., p. 192.

71 E Hay, 'Femininity Tests at the Olympic Games' *Olympic Review*, 76 & 77 (1974), 119-23. 120. The section of the official report of the Mexico Olympiad on the 'Program on Human Genetics and Biology' is illustrated with a karyotype – i.e. a visualisation of the 'normal' chromosomes in an organism. The genetic test for sex used in 1968 was effectively a karyotype test, so it is doubly strange that no connection should be made between the genetic research and sex testing. Indeed, the only mention of sex-chromatin studies is made in a discussion of papers given at the Second International Seminar (pre-Olympics, March 25–29) by Dr Charles E Ford of the UK's 'Atomic Establishments in Harwell' and Dr Oswaldo Forta-Passoa, 'of the University of Sao Paulo. These dealt with chromosome research and stressed the importance of cytological and sex-chromatin studies *when appraised independently of their application to violation of sports regulations* or to intersexuality as the basis for disqualification [my emphasis].' Mexico Organising Committee, *Official Report*, pp. 704–5.

72 [BAS(E)M]. *Annual General Meeting.* 27 Feb. 1953.

73 Ibid.

74 [BAS(E)M] *Minutes of the Executive Committee.* 11 Oct. 1954. This was a notable exception to the rule that most of BAS(E)M's time and attention was spent on adult, elite or professional sports.

75 Anon, 'A Brief History of the Association, with its Aims, and Possible Future Developments' *BJSM* 3 (1968), 143-8.

76 [BAS(E)M] *Minutes of the Executive Committee.* 27 Oct. 1958; Anon, 'A Brief History'.

77 BAS(E)M continued to turn down membership requests from those whose qualifications or professions were judged to be 'medically unacceptable' (mostly osteopaths). [BAS(E)M] *Minutes of the Executive Committee.* 12 Jan. 1968; Anon, 'A Brief History'.

78 [BOA] 34.2 MED INJUR. *Materials on Sports Medicine.* Proceedings of Meetings Held at Loughborough Training College, June 1961, April 1962, June 1963, And a Report by DT Oakley on the Meeting at Goldsmith's College London on the Medical Aspects of Boxing, November 1963. Reprinted from the *Loughborough Journal* 1964.

79 [BAS(E)M] *Report of the Sub-Committee to Consider Problems of Women Athletes,* 27 Apr. 1955.

80 [BAS(E)M] Minutes of the Executive Committee. 1 Dec. 1955.

81 Dr JGP Williams was the registrar in 1959. PH Newman, JPS Thomson, JM Barnes, TCM Moore, 'A Clinic for Athletic Injuries' *Proceedings of the Royal Society of Medicine* 62 (1969), 939-41; [CSSH] SC(RS)(67)17, Appendix A. The Middlesex Hospital Athletes' Clinic; [NA] MH166/1394. *The Sports Council . . .Proposals to Establish Sports Injuries Clinics.* Letter Dr Williams to Mr Philip re. Sports Injuries Clinics, n.d. See Chapter 3 Footnote 120.

82 [BAS(E)M] Minutes of the Executive Committee. 29 Apr. 1957.

83 [BAS(E)M] Annual General Meeting, 26 Feb. 1958; Minutes of the Executive Committee. 8 Apr. 1958.

84 This might, of course, be evidence that such elite athletes were *already* getting specialist treatment elsewhere. Anon, 'Sports Injuries Clinic' *Athletics Weekly* 12.38 (1958). Back cover; [BAS(E)M] *Minutes of the Executive Committee.* 27 Oct. 1958.

85 'Whether we like it or not, national prestige is nowadays frequently measured in terms of prowess of a nation's athletes, and as long as we continue to fail to provide our athletes with first class facilities, be they indoor tracks, new playing fields, gymnasiums and swimming baths, or the best possible care when they are injured or sick, for just so long this country will remain athletically second class.' Anon, 'The Fifth of a Series of Six Articles on the Treatment of Athletic Injuries' *Athletics Weekly* 14.9 (1960), 6-10. 10.

86 Physical Education 55 (1963); [BAS(E)M] *Minutes of the Executive Committee.* 25 Sep. 1968.

87 £2500 was given by the Sports Council, which was matched by the BOA, while other organisations, including the MRC contributed smaller amounts.

Considering this amount as a 'share of GDP', this could be the equivalent of slightly over £100,000 from each organisation, adjusted to 2008 figures. Lawrence H. Officer, 'Five Ways to Compute the Relative Value of a UK Pound Amount, 1830 to Present,' MeasuringWorth, 2008. www.measuring-worth.com/ukcompare/

88  Heggie, 'Only the British'; A Wrynn, '"A Debt Was Paid off in Tears": Science, IOC politics and the Debate about High Altitude in the 1968 Mexico City Olympics' *International Journal of the History of Sport* 23 (2006), 1152-72.

89  J Daniels, 'Altitude and athletic training and performance' *American Journal of Sports Medicine* 7(1979), 371-3. 371.

90  R Bannister, 'The Punishment of a Long Distance Runner' *New York Times Magazine*, 18 Sep. 1966.

91  R Bannister, 'Olympic Games in Mexico – Athletes used as Guinea Pigs' *Times*, 18 Apr. 1966. See also R Bannister, 'A Debt Was Paid Off In Tears: Effects of Altitude on Distance Runners in Mexico' *Sports Illustrated*, 11 Nov. 1968.

92  L Manning, 'The Last Word; I Am Sorry About Mexico's Height' *Daily Mail*, 19 Apr. 1966.

93  Details of the project come from materials in: [BOA] *Medical Committee Box Folder.*

94  British Olympic Association, Report of Medical Research Project into Effects of Altitude in Mexico City in 1965 (London: BOA, 1966).

95  J Coote, 'Olympic Report Attacked' *Telegraph*, 11 Apr. 1966.

96  [BOA] *Medical Committee Box Folder.* Letter KS Duncan to Raymond Owen, 17 Nov. 1967.

97  [CSSH] Appendix G. Sports Council Press Statement, 14 Jul. 1965.

98  [CSSH] SC(RS)(66)8. Research and Statistics Committee (future policy and programme of work), 22 Feb. 1966.

99  [CSSH] Appendix G. Sports Council Press Statement, 14 Jul. 1965.

100  Ibid. For more on training researchers – a topic of interest for the CCPR and the MRC as well – see [NA] CAB124/1646. *Medical Research: Sport.*

101  [CSSH] SC(RS)(66)8a. Preliminary Plans for a Permanent Research Centre for Medicine (paper by Dr O Edholm).

102  On the equipment, see [NA] FD23/4515. *Medical Research and Sport.* Note 'PJC' to Mr Russell, 24 Jun. 1969.

103  [CSSH] SC(RS)(67)15. *Minutes of the Research and Statistics Committee.* General Review Paper, n.d. [c.1967]; SC(RS)(68). *Minutes of the Research and Statistics Committee.* 10 Jan. 1968.

104  [CSSH] SC(RSC)(66)9. *Minutes of the Research and Statistics Committee.* Note of a meeting for the purposes of further discussion of proposals for a Permanent Centre for Sports Medicine, 11 Nov. 1966; SC(RS)(68). *Minutes of the Research and Statistics Committee.* 10 Jan. 1968; SC(RS)(71). *Minutes of the Research and Statistics Committee.* 16 Mar. 1971.

105  See the very extensive report written for the Council by DD Molyneaux: [CSSH] SC(RS)(66)17. *Sports Injuries – A General Background to the Position in Britain.* 25 Aug. 1967.

106 Ibid.
107 Ibid.
108 [CSSH] SC(RS)67. Minutes of the Research and Statistics Committee. 6 Sep. 1967.
109 [CSSH] SC(RS)(68)3. Note of a meeting held at the Ministry of Health on Wednesday 19 November 1967 at 4pm.
110 [CSSH] SC(RS)(69). Minutes of the Research and Statistics Committee. 30 Sep. 1969.
111 [CSSH] SC(RS)(69)18. *Medical Aspects of Sport*, 19 Sep. 1969.
112 [CSSH] ER188/17/4. *Collection of Documents Relating to the European Public Health Committee's Report on the Medical Aspects of Sport* (pub. October 1967). Letter PC McIntosh to DL Skidmore, 26 Feb. 1968.
113 [CSSH] SC(RS)(69) Minutes of the Research and Statistics Committee. 13 May 1968.
114 [CSSH] ER188/17/4. *Collection of Documents.*
115 [CSSH] SC(RS)(69)18. *Medical Aspects of Sport*, 19 Sep. 1969.
116 The Sports Council did not create a working definition of fitness until 1968 when it formed a Fitness Study Group. [CSSH] M.1(G)SC9. *Fitness Study Group.* Report of a Meeting, 30 Sep. 1968.
117 [CSSH] ER188/17/4. *Collection of Documents.* Peter Chisholm McIntosh has written and published widely on sport and society, and his early books are perhaps the first contributions to the history of sport in Britain: see in particular PC McIntosh, *Sport in Society* (London: CA Watts & Co Ltd, 1964) and McIntosh, *Physical Education in England since 1800* (London: G Bell, 1968).
118 J Welshman, 'Only Connect: The History of Sport, Medicine and Society' *International Journal of the History of Sport* 15 (1998), 1–21; Sheard, 'Brutal and Degrading'.
119 JL Blonstein & E Clarke, 'The Medical Aspects of Amateur Boxing' *BMJ* 2 (1954), 1523–5.
120 JW Graham, 'Professional Boxing and the Doctor' *BMJ* 1 (1955), 219–21.
121 [CSSH] SC(RS)(66) Minutes of the Research and Statistics Committee. 26 Sept. 1966.
122 [CSSH] SC(RS)(67) Minutes of the Research and Statistics Committee. 25 Apr. 1967.
123 [CSSH] SC(IR)(72)1 *Terms of Reference*. 27 Oct. 1971.
124 Royal College of Physicians, *Report on the Medical Aspects of Boxing* (London: Royal College of Physicians, 1969).
125 [CSSH] SC(70)6. Report on the Medical Aspects of Boxing, 15 Jan. 1970.
126 Ibid.
127 [CSSH] SC(RS)(70). Minutes of the Research and Statistics Committee. 20 Jan. 1970.
128 [CSSH] SC(IR)(72)1. Terms of Reference, 27 Oct. 1971.
129 Ibid. 'Basic' physiology research is considered to be: the mobile laboratory, an extensive research project into the perception of ball flight, and the bursary to train research students. Grants for 'elite' projects include various

researches into altitude, the boxing study, and research into the detection of anabolic steroids.

130 [CSSH] SC(RS)(68)11. The Institute of Sports Medicine. 26 Feb. 1968.

131 [CSSH] SC(RS)68. Minutes of the Research and Statistics Committee, n.d. c. 1968.

132 [CSSH] SC(RS)(66)17. 'Sports Injuries – A General Background to the Position in Britain'. 25 Aug. 1967.

133 Ibid.

134 Capener was an orthopaedic surgeon, and active in many organisations. See the report of the 'Norman Capener Symposium' organised by the British Orthopaedic Association and the Medical Commission on Accident Prevention, *Annals of the Royal College of Surgeons of England* 57 (1975), 285–95. SB Mostofi (ed.), *Who's Who in Orthopedics* (London: Springer, 2004), 53–6.

135 [BAS(E)M] Minutes of the Executive Committee. 8 Jan. 1969.

136 Ibid.

137 [BAS(E)M] Minutes of the Executive Committee. 24 Sep. 1969.

138 Arthur Charles St John Lawson Johnston, 3rd Baron Luke.

139 [BAS(E)M] Minutes of the Executive Committee. 7 Mar. 1970.

140 Ibid.

141 The Sports Council pointedly took Dr Pugh's side in terms of the 'leaks' to the press; perhaps because Bannister was an ongoing critic of the choice of Mexico City. [CSSH] SC(RS)(67). *Minutes of the Research and Statistics Committee.* 13 Dec. 1967.

142 Jokl, who spent most of his working life in South Africa after fleeing his native Germany, was a founder member of the American College of Sports Medicine and the International Committee for Sport and Physical Education – a wing of UNESCO. [CSSH] SC(RS)(66)25. ICSPE Request for a research committee. 12 Sep. 1966; F Litsky, 'Dr Ernst F Jokl, a Pioneer in Sports Medicine, Dies at 90' *New York Times*, 21 Dec. 1997. See also S Bailey *Science in the Service of Physical Education and Sport: The story of the ICSSPE 1956–1996* (Chichester: John Wiley & Sons, 1996).

143 [CSSH] SC(RS)(66)25. Letter McIntosh to Winterbottom, 19 Dec. 1966. For earlier approaches by Jokl to representatives of British sport and medicine see [NA] FD1/3995. *Research on Athletes and Physical Education, c* 1950.

144 [BOA] *Team Handbooks.* XVII Olympiad, Rome, 1960, p. 10.

145 'The application of psychology is of great importance in the rehabilitation of a player following injury. After a meniscectomy for example, some players need driving, some need leading, many need encouragement, and a few even need restraining.' JE Buck, 'Some Medical Aspects of Team Care at Home' *BJSM* 3 (1968), 121-3. 121.

146 A Porritt, 'Introduction' *Physical Education* 55 (1963), xii.

147 [BOA]. 34.2 MED INJUR. *Materials on Sports Medicine.* Proceedings of Meetings Held at Loughborough Training College, Jun 1961, April 1962, June 1963, and a Report by DT Oakely on the Meeting at Goldsmith's College London on the Medical Aspects of Boxing November 1963.

---

### Box 7. The Olympic medical archive (OMA)

The OMA was the brainchild of the American heart specialist Joseph B Wolffe (d. 1967), one of the founder members of the American College of Sports Medicine. In 1960 he was the vice-president of FIMS, and together with the General Secretary (Guiseppe La Cava) developed proposals for the creation of an Olympic Medical Archive. Wolffe convinced both the IOC and the World Health Organization that these archives would be useful; the aim was to collect extensive physiological data on Olympic competitors, which would be updated every four years for the lifetime of the athletes involved. These records would be deposited in the Olympic Museum in Lausanne, Switzerland. The physiological data could be correlated with athletic performance, and with their general medical records and causes of death. The language of the archives is hyperbolic – the introductory paragraph on the inside cover of the proposal document issued in June 1963 reads 'Let us not overlook Acres of Diamonds within our reach ... [these records will leave] a heritage to benefit the health of future generations. It will be another victory for the human spirit'.

Physiological tests were supposed to take place in the athletes' home countries, and a standardised booklet was produced for examiners to fill in. These tests were incredibly extensive, as the original booklet was A3, with fourteen pages to record test results, and it even had slots on the back for x-ray prints. FIMS recommended that every country with an Olympic organisation ought to produce a sub-committee just to deal with the Archives.

Testing did take place in 1964 in advance of the Games in Tokyo, although the organisers were disappointed by the relatively low return of forms (1121 of about 5000). This was despite the promise of certificates, possibly even some sort of medal, and the honorary title of 'Volunteer for Science' for the athletes who did participate. Surveying was carried out for the 1968 games in Mexico, and the extensive forms were simplified in the hope of increasing returns. But athletes were unwilling to take the time and effort to participate in testing, and sporting organisations and governments were unwilling to find the money and resources for such extensive testing and experimentation.

With the death of Wolffe in 1967 the scheme lost its major promoter, and was unable to overcome its difficulties and the resistance of participants. No testing took place in 1972, or at any subsequent games.

See:
[BOA] 34.2 MED INJUR. *Materials on Sports Medicine,*. 34.20 The Olympic Medical Archives – A Proposal; 34.23, Report of the Olympic Medical Archives, Tokyo 1964 (ed. Toshiro Azuma); 34.24 report of the Olympic Medical Archives, Mexico 1968.

Anon, 'Obituary: Dr Joseph Wolffe (President of the OMA)' *Bulletin du Comite International Olympique* 97 (1967), 35.

V Heggie 'Volunteers for Science: Medicine, Health and the Modern Olympic Games' in V. Nutton (ed.) *Sport, Medicine and Immortality* (British Museum, forthcoming)

## Box 8. Dr Lewis Griffiths Cresswell Evans Pugh (1909–94)

Dr LGCE Pugh is probably better known for his work on some of the major scientific expeditions of the twentieth century, both to altitude and the Antarctic, than his contributions to sports medicine. Qualifying with a medical degree from Oxford in 1939 he joined the army, and began a lifetime's work on physiology at the Mountain Warfare Training Centre where he worked with ski troops.

After World War II, Pugh briefly conducted research in rheumatology and cardiovascular physiology, before being invited on his first major expedition in 1947, accompanying a British Naval voyage to the Arctic Circle. In 1950, after working as a house physician at Hammersmith Hospital in London he was appointed to the Medical Research Council's Human Physiology Division where he remained for much of his career.[1] While continuing to work on extreme physiology – the body's reaction to high and low temperatures, to cold immersion, exhaustion and low oxygen pressure – he also consulted for and travelled with several major expeditions, including three major Himalayan trips (including the famous 1960–61 Silver Hut expedition) and the 1957 Trans-Arctic Expedition.[2]

Pugh is credited with ensuring the success of Norgay and Hillary's ascent of Everest in 1953; he was a medical consultant for the trip and calculated the necessary supplies of both oxygen and fresh water. It was his experience not only in physiology, but also in active mountaineering which allowed him on to the 1968 Mexican Research Trip; throughout the 1970s he continued to use athletes as guinea pigs in his research into endurance and the effects of temperature.

[1] JB West, *High Life: A History of High-Altitude Physiology and Medicine* (Oxford: Oxford University Press, 1998), pp. 269–73. See also footnote 5, Chapter 10.
[2] J Milledge, 'Obituaries: Griffith Pugh' *Independent*, 27 Jan. 1995.

### Box 9. John GP Williams (1932–95)

As the author of the first British text on sports medicine, published in 1962, Williams epitomised the interdisciplinary nature of the specialty. From Cambridge he went to St Mary's hospital in London, qualifying in 1956; to this he added one diploma in obstetrics and gynaecology, and one in physical medicine, became a Fellow of the Royal College of Surgeons, and gained an MSc in 'spinal mechanisms':

> 'he . . . became a physician who operated, a very unusual and perhaps lonely situation. He pioneered several surgical procedures for soft tissue injuries and more recently was used a great deal for medico legal and compensation advice.'[1]

Partly through his interest in rehabilitation, and partly through connections forged by his wife, Sally Williams (a physiotherapist), Williams worked as a senior registrar at the Middlesex Hospital (which had the UK's first sports injuries clinic – see Chapter 3), as a consultant at Mount Vernon Hospital, and also as a consultant at Stoke Mandeville, home of the Paralympics (see Chapter 3).[2] Eventually he settled at Farnham Park Rehabilitation Centre, where he was appointed director in 1965. Farnham Park offered general rehabilitative treatment for NHS patients, but also maintained second 'stream' of patients with athletic injuries.[3] As well as pioneering treatments, particularly for soft tissue injuries, Farnham Park also functioned as an important training ground for the next generation of sports medics.[3]

In addition to his role as teacher, and his seminal textbook *Sports Medicine*, Williams was a significant figure in institutional terms, both at the national and international level. He was the secretary of BAS(E)M between 1962 and 1973, and of FIMS for a decade from 1970.[1] His involvement with sports medicine organisations diminished in the 1980s, partly due to an ongoing dispute with a colleague whose career he had shaped, Dr Peter Sperryn.[1,2]

[1] DT Pedoe, 'Obituary: Dr John GP Williams' *BJSM* 29 (1995), 220–2.
[2] LA Reynolds and EM Tansey (eds), *The Development of Sports Medicine in Twentieth Century Britain* (London: Wellcome Trust, 2009); particularly the evidence of Sally Williams and Dr Peter Sperryn and p. 130.
[3] PA Fricker, 'Sports medicine training in England' *Australian Journal of Sports Medicine* 13 (1981), 43–4.

# 5

# Sport for All and the inert majority, 1970–87

In 1987, nearly three decades after the founding of the British Olympic Association's first Medical Committee, the British Olympic Medical Centre was opened at Northwick Park Hospital. Its opening symbolises the full institutionalisation of elite, specialist sports medicine. Given that the last chapter described the self-creation of sports medicine as a discipline which focused on just these sorts of bodies, the opening of this centre should come as no surprise. But the dominant theme of this chapter is rather the provision of this sort of specialist and expert treatment to the lay, public body, not to the elite athlete. In a traditional story about professions or medical specialties, the opening of special interest clinics would be a positive sign for sports medicine, indicating official and institutional recognition not only of the theoretical grounding but also the practical need for specialism. But sports medicine is not a typical medical specialty and in fact the promotion of Sports Injuries Clinics (SICs) was a direct threat to the expertise and self-identity of sports medicine practitioners in Britain. These clinics symbolised a real challenge to the very justification for sports medicine – the athletic body as a discrete medical object.

Although the leisure revolution of the 1970s was not quite as dramatic as promised (the leisure boom of the 1960s being curtailed by economic problems in the early '70s), rising personal wealth did lead to an increased participation in sport, athletics and exercise in leisure time.[1] This was added to by increasing state intervention in sport, through the Sports Council and other organisations, an emergent public health drive to encourage exercise, and European interventions. The increases in participation were not limited to traditional team sports or games, but included the 5 and 10 kilometre run, the marathon, and new high-intensity sports such as squash. One sports doctor described this (in 1986) as 'an epidemic of sport', clearly requiring medical intervention.[2]

The catchphrase which underpinned much of this development was 'Sport for All'. First adopted by the Council of Europe around 1966, and promoted through the International Council of Sport and Physical

Education (part of UNESCO) in the 1970s, Sport for All was a blanket term used for a variety of purposes by governments, public health activists, the media, doctors and sports organisations.[3] In the last chapter I discussed how a related report from the Council of Europe, *The Medical Aspects of Sport*, was dismissed in Britain, in part because its concept of sports medicine did not match that being produced nationally. Sport for All also posed a direct challenge to the athletic body which British sports medicine by now regarded as the proper subject and object of its gaze, by reconsidering what 'sport' meant:

> The concept of Sport for All – which is quite different from the traditional conception of sport – embraces not only sport proper but also, and perhaps above all, various forms of physical activity, from spontaneous unorganised games to a minimum of physical exercise regularly performed.[4]

In the preceding chapter we saw how sports doctors and other sports professionals had successfully described the athlete's body as special and abnormal. In doing so they had interpreted sport as a 'professional' activity – i.e. one requiring training, specific equipment, physiological adaptations in the body, and so on. Yet in the 1970s and 1980s the focus (at least in terms of finance and political support) seemed to be shifting away from the elite performer, and back towards community sport, physical education, and the general body of the public. This was probably the first time that the government in Britain had taken such a close interest in the physical activity of its electorate in peace time, or at least without direct connections to the fitness of a population upon which military strength depended.

It is not the purpose of this chapter (or this book) to explain in detail why there was a renewed interest in national fitness, but I would suggest that two factors played a central role. On the one hand there is the leisure revolution itself, increasing popular demand for, and interest in, the provision of sports and exercise facilities. On the other is the 'new public health', as described by Berridge and others, which focused on interventionist approaches to lifestyle – that is, the role of smoking, drinking, diet and exercise (and illegal drugs) on the health costs of the nation. Elsewhere this has been characterised as the rise of the 'risk-factor'.[5] What all of these issues have in common is that an analysis of their costs and consequences requires quite sophisticated epidemiological and statistical work. To the suspicion that exercise could kill was gradually added evidence that it might also cure, a balance which poses difficult (and still unresolved) questions about state responsibility for encouraging healthy lifestyles while at the same time dealing with the medical consequences of increased sporting activity.[6]

In this new medico-political atmosphere British sports medicine, as an emergent specialism, faced two direct threats. On the one hand, the Sport for All movement and the opening of SICs threatened to normalise sporting activity, and through that subsume sports treatment, training and even policing within other established specialties. It is deeply significant that the early SICs were hospital-based and often surgeon-run, while BAS(E)M was largely populated by general practitioners and other primary care professionals. There was a possibility that the athletic body might be dissolved as a clinical entity, removing any justification for sports medicine as a discrete form of medical knowledge. On the other hand, if sports doctors maintained a strict line on the uniqueness of the elite athlete, they risked total abstraction from general health care, essentially limiting themselves to a tiny patient pool of physiologically abnormal human specimens, with little relevance to the NHS.

This challenge was practical as well as theoretical. To get money for specialist sports medicine activities it was necessary to prove that sport had special, *additional* medical needs; yet by highlighting the potential risks of sport, the rewards of sport as a health-giving activity could be undermined, cutting off potential funding gained from public health sources. There is no doubt, too, that the assumptions of sports medicine professionals – that athletes were different and deserved special treatment – were not shared by everyone in the wider medical, scientific or political community. As a medical adviser to the Department of Health and Social Security (DHSS) wrote around 1971: 'I would personally give priority to a window cleaner with a sprained ankle sustained at work over a bank clerk with a similar injury that occurred in a football match on Saturday afternoon'.[7]

How did the individuals and organisations which made up British sports medicine deal with these threats? By using a rhetoric of sport as a *drug* or *disease*. The quote above about an 'epidemic' of sport is indicative – increasingly we see the language of medicine applied directly to sport and physical activity, so that by the end of the 1980s we see exercise regularly described as a drug, with doctors discussing an 'exercise prescription', or even the 'side-effects' of exercise.[8] Sports medicine did not resolve the dichotomy between the athletic body and the lay body; instead it sought to bridge the gap with its professional expertise. If anything, the divide between the super/abnormal athlete and the fit layman increased – by 1988 there was nothing particularly controversial in a doctor suggesting that '[i]t is fair to state that most sportsmen are not healthy', and that rather than being 'fit', they were 'fit for purpose'.[9] Sports and games were conceptualised as *specialist* activities which required careful preparation and even physiological adaptation before the normal person could safely take part in them. Sports governing bodies, even those advocating Sport for All, were careful to advise new devotees to 'get fit to play sports' rather than 'play sports to get fit'.[10] So while the body of the elite athlete was increasingly rarefied, now the body of the lay sportsman was co-opted into an interpretation of physical activity which required special advice and professional knowledge.

While trends in leisure habits and sports policy could undermine the intellectual basis of the specialism, more practical threats to prestige, authority, even membership fees, were emerging. Relations between all the organisations founded in the last chapter became strained at the end of the century, which is illustrated here by the conflicts over SICS and various sports medicine centres. These clinics were in turn affected by broader political and economic trends, as some closed down in the early 1980s as a consequence of more general Thatcherite crackdowns on public spending, while a booming market in part-private sports injuries clinics in the mid-1970s was regularly threatened by Barbara Castle who disliked what she considered two-tier systems in the NHS.[11]

But the most significant thing about the SICs was that by-and-large they were not related to BAS(E)M, still the leading sports medicine organisation. Instead many were started as part of a scheme by the Sports Council, which excluded most BAS(E)M members. Further, the definition of 'sports medicine' embodied by this practice was narrowly conceived, subservient to other healthcare demands, embedded in hospitals and not run by specialists – a model which clearly undermined the attempts by both BAS(E)M and the Institute of Sports Medicine to produce a rigorous, academically respected science of a new sort of body.[12] In addition there was a proliferation of (often private) sports medicine centres, run by both doctors and auxiliary medical professionals such as physiotherapists. Some of these were set up by individuals who were not recognised as experts by BAS(E)M, leading to calls for systems to 'officially' recognise who was a sports medicine expert, and who was, to use their own language, just a 'quack' running a 'back-street clinic'.[13]

So alongside the debates over SICs and other sports medicine centres was an ongoing and intertwined debate about sports medicine as a specialty. Initially many in BAS(E)M still resisted the idea that sports medicine needed to be recognised formally as a medical specialty in Britain, but gradually the organisation's official line (at least as represented in the *British Journal of Sports Medicine* and its editorials) began to shift towards actively campaigning for recognition. For nearly all sports medics *some* sort of formal recognition became an imperative – if not full specialist accreditation, then at least proper certification, courses, and eventually postgraduate education schemes. Sports medicine was closing ranks; its expertise could no longer be policed and maintained by a gentleman's agreement, an understanding about expertise and experience, it now needed to be proved to outside bodies, and protected from them, with paper certificates and even licenses.

Sometimes this protectionism was justified using the bodies of their patients. After all, if athletes were different, if they were special, then they needed specialist expert advice – not normal medical care from inexperienced generalists. Significantly, too, now the *lay* body also needed protecting; risk and responsibility were key issues in the late 1970s and 1980s. Who was responsible if a runner were to have a heart attack while taking part in one of the dozens of new charity fun runs? Non-fatal injuries could prove even more difficult; doctors were often accused of considering sporting injuries to be essentially self-inflicted, and therefore less 'worthy' of treatment – yet when the government itself was encouraging its population to exercise more, did it not have a moral obligation to provide health care for sports injuries? The possibility of being involved in legal disputes (although generally not seen in the UK until the 1990s) also made apparent the need for certification, so that 'experts' could be readily identified and asked to give testimony.[14]

## Sports medicine for all?

Sport was a double edged sword. While it had potential (and the research evidence for this was growing) to deliver social, financial and public health benefits, when used wrongly it could cause sickness, injury, disease and even death – and these messages were widely spread in the public sphere through the popular media.[15] The institutions of British sports medicine promoted the idea that the only way to successfully use sport as a tool for health was through the guidance of specialists; one got exercise 'on prescription' in the same way one got any other drug, from a qualified medical expert. The caution about sport which some historians see in the late nineteenth century is possibly better placed in late twentieth. Most organisations and individuals (particularly the Department or Ministry of Health) were initially wary of promoting physical exercise on the grounds of health, considering any connections weak or unproven. Even where exercise was considered health giving, there was still much debate in this period about how much and what sort of exercise should be done. Once again, vulnerable groups – women, children, patients with heart disease – were particularly highlighted for specialist, cautionary, advice.[16]

European-style policing in sport, such as the sort of interventionalist programme recommended by *Medical Aspects of Sport* and rejected so firmly by the Sports Council in the 1960s, was now being actively mobilised to reaffirm sports medicine's position as a specialty. It is particularly notable in the coverage of increasingly popular marathon and fun run events.[17] For example – in 1984 the Sports Council's Fitness and Health Advisory Group collaborated with the Health Education Council to write a set of guidelines for the organisation of, and participation in, British marathons and half-marathons.[18] These guidelines are extremely comprehensive, covering some issues that might not immediately appear to be directly relevant to sports medicine, including how to avoid the risk of trampling at the start, and how and why a race ought to be cancelled. Heavy emphasis is placed on the need for expert or experienced staff, and it is clearly stated that a *doctor* ought to be recruited onto the organising body as soon as possible, not 'just' medical auxiliaries.[19] Further, this advice is not just about treatment and emergency care, but also concerns itself with enhancement; standardised handouts for would-be participants were devised, which covered issues from clothing though pre-race training to dietary advice.

The diet of the athlete received renewed interest in the 1970s and 1980s. As a reflection of the shift in the athletic body the recommended diet had already changed from a 'normal' healthy diet to something more specialised. While mainstream medicine eschewed the possibility of wonderfoods after the early claims for vitamins, relatively physiologically complex systems of eating were promoted for all would-be athletes. Carbohydrate loading, which involves fasting and then feasting on complex carbohydrates to 'load' glycogen stores in the muscle, rose to prominence in the 1970s and is still widely used today. Of course, what was suitable for the elite athlete was not necessarily good for the new body of the lay athlete – the leaflets for runners discussed above explicitly dismiss carbohydrate loading for 'amateur' marathoners, and there were concerns voiced about the safety of athletic dietary schemes over the long term, or in vulnerable bodies (still broadly interpreted to mean anyone who was not young, fit and male).[20]

Dietary supplements had long been aimed at sportsmen and women, and in the 1970s and 1980s the traditional products of dextrose tablets, Horlicks, and Oxo were increasingly competing against sophisticated glucose drinks, protein powders, and other commercial sports products. The pages of the *British Journal of Sports Medicine* were opened to adverts in the mid-1970s; at first these tended towards pharmaceutical products, notably analgesics and massage gels, but the first 'performance drink' appears in the early 1980s. Such products (and home-made alternatives) were the subject of many experiments; between 1971 and 1973 three articles on the uses of glucose drinks were published in the *British Journal of Sports Medicine* alone.[21] The advertising of these products is often aspirational, so while sports medicine may have been telling the layperson that they could, or should, not achieve an athletic body (at least not without extraordinary dedication), since the nineteenth century advertisers had been suggesting that sporting glory could be bought for the price of a tub of cocoa or an energy bar.[22]

Everywhere in sports medicine appears this desire to bridge the gap between the lay and the elite athlete, and to allow the lay person access to the apparent expertise of the sports medic. 1970, the start date for this chapter, is particularly significant for British sports medicine, as in September of that year the 18th World Congress of Sports Medicine was held in Oxford – the first time this meeting had gathered in the UK. In his opening address Eldon Griffiths (b. 1925), the Minister with special responsibility for sport, argued that:

> The international sportsman, the first-class football and athletics clubs all have the benefits of modern science and medicine at their behest. That is as it should be. But we need the benefit of this experience and expertise at every level of sporting activity, just as we need the collective wisdom of everyone engaged in sports medicine right down at grass roots level.[23]

It was this extension of expertise from the elite to the lay athlete, even to the realm of public health and exercise for sport, which drove the institutional and intellectual changes in sports medicine over this period.

Griffiths' characterisation of the medical care for elite athletes is somewhat idealised; there was still plenty of debate and complaint about the treatment of international and national-level sportsmen and women between 1970 and 1987 (and beyond). Examples are easy to find; while research was undertaken into new treatments for soft tissue injuries, including the use of proteolytic enzymes and corticosteroid injections, they were not universally offered in practice.[24] Even the balance between rest and exercise as healing processes became controversial again; in 1972 Dr Elizabeth Ferris, ex-Olympic diver and expert in nutrition, wrote an article in *Sports World* which was picked up by the *Times*, complaining that:

> The usual advice that an injured athlete will get from the average doctor is to rest – the medical panacea for all ills, but there are many Olympic medallist who would never have climbed the victory rostrum if they had followed the conservative dictum.[25]

It is also worth pointing out that although by the 1970s most sports seem to have appointed medical officers, and gone some way to formalising their medical support, this was often still dependent on voluntary services, and varied considerably according to the local context and the availability of local enthusiasts and sympathetic medical professionals. A case in point would be the 4th European Youth Swimming and Diving Championships, held in Leeds in August 1973. The medical services at this event were extensive, and yet still reliant on voluntary service and the good will of private organisations and institutions. A 'generous list of drugs' was provided free by Boots Ltd., in exchange for 'a prominent acknowledgement in the programme'; a sixteen-bedded sick bay was provided and staffed largely by volunteers, some of whom were using their own annual leave in order to attend; diagnostic and physiotherapeutic services, and even some furnishings, were sourced from the local hospital, which was one of only a half-dozen or so in the country to happen to have an established sports injuries service.[26] Thus, competitors at the games had access to specialist sports injuries treatment and diagnosis both at the poolside and in a hospital setting. They received laboratory, clinical, diagnostic and even prescribing services for free. Their coaches and trainers had access to a co-ordinating Medical Officer with expertise in sports medicine and swimming. It is therefore quite possible – in fact it was the norm – for a highly specialised and professional service to be provided *voluntarily.*

The theme of greater access to sports medicine is echoed in the fact that provision in the field had clearly moved beyond the 'field', beyond the track, football ground and boxing ring, to the pool, stadia and on courts. Indeed, in 1976 the mainstream medical journal, the *Practitioner* – a publication aimed mostly at the general practitioner or family doctor – carried an article by the Medical Officer to the British Everest Expedition on 'the care of the mountaineer' which contained advice and guidance for athletic and lay bodies alike. The advice he gave was for everyone from the 'member of a weekend school walking party in North Wales ... [to] an expedition of several months' duration to the Himalayas'.[27] Such immediate care was a resurgent interest for those involved with sports medicine; this is in part connected with the increasing popularity of marathons and fun runs, but was also a consequence of the gradual televisation of sports. Errors of judgement on the pitch or track could be 'watched by millions'.[28] Doctors now had the opportunity to comment on the principles and organisation of first-aid treatment even at events they had not attended, and the fact that these events were so publicly visible meant that they could be considered opportunities to educate the population (and, conversely, were a dangerous advert for poor or inappropriate treatment techniques).

The media coverage of athletes' injuries could also lead to increasing demand for sports services from the general public, as they diagnosed themselves with the conditions of their sporting heroes, or echoed Eldon Griffiths' sentiment that these specialist services should be available to all. The burgeoning of private SICs (there were over thirty in the UK by 1986) suggests a reasonable amount of patient demand.[29] SICs had opened in Britain as early as the 1940s, although these were usually temporal rather than physical clinics – a special slot on Monday mornings or Sunday afternoons in some other clinic or A&E department. These clinics were not necessarily formally recognised by their local management or the DHSS, and were, as a sports doctor wrote in 1975, 'ghost clinics'.[30] Some clinics focused on elite athletes; the Human Performance Laboratory at Salford University had been formed in the late 1960s, and by 1974 was offering an '"ad hoc" service to sportsmen, including Olympic wrestlers, athletes, cyclists and swimmers, professional soccer players and international netball and tennis players'.[31] This service was laboratory-based, and offered diagnostics, some treatment and advice, although 'because of the limited funds that could be withdrawn from [their] own budget for such work, [they did] not publicise [their] service'.[32]

As well as Salford's laboratory, the physiology/sports science departments at Loughborough and at Birmingham were key academic players, applying to both the Sports Council and the MRC for grants.[33] Most such centres provided dope and gender testing, physiological measurement for the design of training and rehabilitation schemes and some direct medical intervention. Even universities without such sports-orientated laboratories provided facilities, which could be available for local and amateur sportsmen as well as the elite athlete. In 1978 '[w]ith financial support from the Boots Company Ltd.' – because the Department of Health had refused financial assistance – Manchester University's Student Health Centre and Department of Orthopaedic Surgery co-operated to create a SIC.[34] This clinic operated four times a week, with staff from the Department and a full time physiotherapist, and there was a 'treatment room in the University indoor sports complex with access to a small gymnasium, multi-gym, large sports hall and swimming pool'.[35] Although the original intention was to provide a clinic for students and staff this soon expanded to the treatment of athletes belonging to local clubs, and also those listed by the North West 'Centre of Excellence'.[36] Despite some successes, including at least one former patient who gained a place at the 1980 Olympics, the clinic was threatened with closure in 1982 due to the reforms in academic funding implemented by the Thatcher government.

The Institute of Sports Medicine made a notable (and for this organisation, relatively rare) contribution to the practical provision of medical care to athletes by enabling the foundation of a sports clinic in Cambridge. In 1978 Dr Sylvia Lachmann was appointed as the first Sports Medicine Fellow, sponsored by the Institute, at New Hall – now Murray Edwards College – Cambridge. Subsequently she and Sir John Butterfield (1920–2000), then Master of Downing College, collaborated to form a sports clinic at Addenbrooke's Hospital that would provide diagnosis, treatment and advice to student athletes, as well as acting as a centre for research (particularly into soft tissue injuries). Funding was sourced from the University, the Institute, and from the *Daily Mirror*; the clinic still exists and is named after Peter Wilson, a *Mirror* sports writer.[37]

For most SICs the primary concern was the treatment of injuries and disabilities (and for the Sports Council's clinics, the reporting of sports injuries). Those which aimed to treat the elite athlete, or were based in a university setting, tended to also focus on issues of enhancement and policing. For example, the Manchester University clinic concentrated on treatment and rehabilitation, but it also allowed physiologists and physicians to practise sports medicine as a research activity. Those who offered their time (for free) at these clinics gained access to human guinea pigs and testing facilities, and did produce publishable research.[38] Manchester's clinic also shows the keen interest of the commercial sector in sports medicine; Boots has been a recurrent name in the sponsorship of British sports medicine since their involvement with the 1948 London Olympics. By 1986, in addition to other SICs, there were over a dozen private physiotherapy clinics offering specialist services to sportsmen and women. Some nominally 'private' clinics were actually run within NHS facilities by NHS staff – often asking for 'a trivial fee or for a donation to sports medicine research funds'.[39]

So sports medicine for the elite practitioner was still largely provided voluntarily, yet some sports medicine for the lay body was becoming a profit-making enterprise – at least for a few dozen private injuries and sports medicine clinics. The growth of the commercial sector contributed directly to moves towards formalising sports medicine's specialty status, and did so in two ways. Firstly, BAS(E)M, the Institute of Sports Medicine, and other representatives of established sports medicine interest in Britain sought to regain control over who was and who was not able to call themselves an 'expert' in sports medicine to eliminate the 'quacks' and 'backstreet clinics'. Secondly, however, the relatively precarious position of private practice meant that those who did run such sports injuries clinics were themselves often keen on formal recognition for their expertise.

In the late 1970s and early 1980s some sports doctors found themselves in conflict with health insurance companies precisely because they were not practitioners of a formal specialism. One insurance company wrote to Dr Malcolm Read (sometime Medical Officer to the BOA) in 1984 to say that:

> the Underwriters, whom we represent, specify that a patient claiming benefit under the terms of their policies of insurance should have been treated, or had their treatment supervised, by someone who holds, or has held, an appointment of consultant status at a NHS Hospital.[40]

These conditions could prevent their subscribers claiming any payouts for specialist treatment in sports medicine, which had no NHS consultancies. While individual doctors managed to renegotiate the terms of their contracts –with many insurance companies recognising sports medicine as an exception to this rule – the possibility of a threat to their income continued as policies and procedures were reviewed through the 1980s and 1990s.

Some recognition could be achieved by completing a course in sports medicine, and these proliferated in the 1970s and 1980s. In the late 1960s BAS(E)M had started to run 'summer schools', week long courses in sports medicine at Loughborough, and in 1975 these were restructured and formally recognised by FIMS (making attendees eligible to join the international society).[41] The British Postgraduate Medical Federation, representing postgraduate medical students, specifically requested in 1975 that BAS(E)M should endeavour to continue to provide these courses at least annually. In 1974 special education went further, when the Conjoint Board (dually representing the Royal Colleges of Physicians and of Surgeons) added Sports Medicine as a special option to Part II of its Diploma in Medical Rehabilitation.[42] This was followed in the early 1980s by a Diploma in Sports Medicine at the London Hospital organised by the Institute of Sports Medicine, and then one based at the (BAS(E)M-organised) London Sports Medicine Institute, founded in 1986.[43] Opportunities for formal training in areas outside of, and affiliated to, medicine also increased – particularly in connection to the university centres discussed above.[44]

### Rehabilitation and risk

The practice of sports medicine has become diverse and complex, as has its site of provision. Its practitioners, however, are increasingly easy to recognise – they are members of sports medicine organisations, hold certificates and other qualifications, and are recognised by other bodies. (Dr Hugh Burry was appointed as the first Honorary Consultant in Sports Medicine to the Sports Council in 1975).[45] Most notably, however, its patient group was now not just the athletic body, but also the body public. Sports medicine gained access to the lay body either because individuals actively sought out specialist treatment (as evidenced by the private SICs) or through a rhetoric of risk. Sport was a drug which required practitioner control – used correctly it could cure, used incorrectly it could kill. This tension was perhaps most notable in one resurgent area of sports medicine treatment, and that is the use of sport as a rehabilitative treatment.

Rehabilitation through sport had been ongoing since Guttman's work in the 1940s, but the 1970s and 1980s saw a particular interest in the use of vigorous exercise for the rehabilitation of patients with heart disease. Despite initial anxiety about the safety of vigorous exercise for post-coronary patients and 'at risk' groups both the MRC and the Sports Council eventually agreed to fund one large-scale study on 'the effects of exercise in middle-aged men' in the early 1970s.[46] The Sports Council's total funding of £7500 to this project made it the largest single grant paid to date, and it remained the largest such grant until the end of the decade.[47] This form of exercise was even more explicitly a drug, or a medication – tailored for the individual, heavily supervised and effectively given 'on prescription'.[48]

Risk is also central to dialogues about enhancement. Altitude, for example, was reinvented as a training regime, rather than a threat to the health of athletes. The BOA arranged for some members of the British Olympic Team – rowing, canoeing, pentathlon, and some of the athletics team – to undergo a three week altitude training programme before the Munich Games in 1972 (any pretence that the British Olympian competed as a pure amateur without specialist assistance had by now disappeared). The results of this trip 'showed a significant improvement in performance', but there were still disagreements about how much of this improvement was physiological and how much psychological.[49] Of the ten international teams training at St Moritz at the same time one (the USA) thought altitude training had been unhelpful, six thought it was physiological, and two thought it to be purely psychological, with one team uncertain about what caused the improved performance.

Some other long-running controversies about risk also came to a head. After the ambivalent reports on the health effects of boxing published by BAS(E)M in the mid-1960s and by the Royal College of Physicians in 1969, debates over the safety and morality of boxing – both professional and amateur – continued in the medical press. Surveys and case studies added weight to the proposal that boxing was too dangerous to be considered a legitimate leisure activity. In 1982 the Annual Meeting of the British Medical Association passed a resolution 'that, in view of the proven ocular and brain damage resulting from professional boxing, the association should campaign for its abolition'.[50] BAS(E)M and its members maintained their ambivalent position, however:

> [t]he medical risks of amateur boxing are few, and even professional boxing is much more strictly controlled from a medical point of view . . . The moral issue, of whether it is permissible to allow people to participate in a sport whose main objective is to inflict injury upon another, is less clearly defined.[51]

Sports medicine was therefore distinct. Its organisations could hold contrary views to mainstream representatives of British medicine. It could be found in specialist clinics as well as on the field, by the pool and (controversially) in the ring. Its practitioners may well have completed courses, and by 1987 could hold diplomas and certificates. It was of political importance, and full of 'politics'. For the first time sports medics had to emphasise enhancement and policing as core parts of their activity, as treatment was in danger of being subsumed into regular soft tissue and orthopaedic treatment within the NHS. But for the first time, too, it began to seem important to use sports medicine experts to treat the lay, as well as the athletic body.

## The Olympics and international sports medicine

This increasing number of medical personnel with certificates or diplomas in sports medicine, or who claimed other evidence of expert knowledge in the field, was not limited to Britain. When the organising committee of the 1972 Munich Games advertised for volunteers to take up medical positions, 1197 individuals applied for just 225 available positions. It was the German and Bavarian Associations of Sport who had the final say in who was selected for these voluntary posts, and they were able to be choosy in their selection, applying a broad range of criteria. As well as being relatively young and fit, candidates also had to prove that they had knowledge and experience in the care of athletes, specific experience of sports medicine, and ideally a proficiency in several languages.[52] In the extensive three-floor Olympic Hospital there were surgical and x-ray facilities, as well as rooms equipped for internal medicine specialists. These, and the many first aid and local medical clinics, were staffed by the Red Cross, the Armed Forces and volunteers from the University of Munich, as well as the final list of 225 'qualified' volunteers. Munich reflects well the trend to specialisation and specialism; the medical services for spectators were treated (in the administration of the Games and in the report) entirely separately to those for the athletes.

Although the IOC set limits on the numbers of team members (including doctors) who could travel with the competitors, this was as much due to security restrictions as to a desire to make team support equal across nations.[53] Consequently nothing stopped teams from taking multiple practitioners (as many as they could find and afford), just so long as they remained outside the Olympic Village. For Munich the British team took a Chief Medical Officer (Owen) and three Medical Officers (Drs R Kennedy, W Mitchell and M Read) as well as a Chief Physiotherapist, and two assistant Physiotherapists.[54] By 1976 (Montreal) an additional physiotherapist and masseur were (officially) added to the team, while the yachting team took their own doctor and the cyclists brought a joint coach/masseur.[55]

The report for Montreal is the first which directly mentions the centralisation of dope and gender testing, and gives some detail on the organisation of the process, which involved specialist medical teams whose only duty was to perform the 2001 tests carried out.[56] Elsewhere, over 1000 medical-related staff treated nearly 10,000 athletic patients, although interestingly the Organising Committee felt that the establishment of the polyclinic (effectively the Village hospital) was a 'needless expense'.[57] They argued that the local medical facilities in any major metropolitan centre were sufficient for any serious medical needs beyond first aid, so long as they were properly co-ordinated. The Committee also played down the role of locally provided medical advice, tipping the balance in favour of the doctors who travelled with the nations' teams; they stated that local doctors should always be deferential in favour of the team doctor when it came to questions about when and whether an injured player should return to training or compete (this deference did not apply, of course, in the case of failed dope or gender tests). It is clear that by this point most teams were bringing many medical professionals with them who were able to deal with the majority of training questions, dietary problems, rehabilitation requirements and minor injuries and illnesses.

The British team took yet more support to Moscow in 1980. The medical team was supplemented with an additional physiotherapist, while the athletics, cycling, Judo, and swimming teams all brought various extra medical team members.[58] The Team Handbook for this year reveals deep-seated concerns about the services at the (politically sensitive) Moscow Olympics: '[i]t is suggested by many sources that the sanitary and hygiene arrangements may not be entirely satisfactory at all venues in Moscow'.[59] Athletes were advised to avoid unbottled water, 'highly spiced dishes', ice-cream, and so on. Likewise, team members were strongly advised not to attend the proposed 'physiological testing station', 'without the agreement of their team doctor or team manager, or without approaching one of the HQ Medical Team first'.[60] Even more forcefully, the Handbook states that 'under no circumstances should any competitor attend the Polyclinic, except in cases of emergency, without the agreement of their team doctor'.[61] It is unclear why athletes should avoid the clinic (which in Moscow was a reduced version of the Village hospital, effectively just an outpatients department), although with regard to the Dispensary the Handbook also gives a dire warning: '[i]f in doubt at any time as to whether any medicament contains 'Dope' of any kind, come and ask one of the Team Doctors BEFORE taking it'.[62]

The actual purpose of the 'physiological testing station' is not entirely clear. The Official Report of the Moscow Games claims that this was the 'first' time such testing had taken place, which is clearly untrue in light of the Olympic Medical Archive activity in the 1960s and other research which had taken place at previous games. The clinic;

> [i]ncorporated a sports testing and functional diagnostics section equipped with running tracks, bicycle ergometers, gas analysers and instruments for biochemical and detailed cardiological tests. Here the athletes could check their fitness and consult specialists.[63]

Demand seems high for the more regular medical services, as about 5000 athletes sought treatment, although some of this was just the prescription of pharmaceuticals. Supply was also high; the Organising Committee ended up providing almost one doctor and more than one nurse for every injured athlete – 4176 physicians and 5248 nurses, with nearly 1000 'sanitary epidemiologists' (although these figures are probably inflated, like those of Tokyo in 1964, through the secondment of local medical services and associated staff).

As well as the Polyclinic there were also a series of special clinics and emergency services to convey injured athletes to beds and wards at local hospitals and medical research facilities. All this was in line with the IOC's own rules on medical services, which by the 1980s had expanded massively from their initial recommendation, accepted in the 1910s, that the marathon should be run in the coolest part of the day. Reports from the Moscow Games strongly emphasised that the medical arrangements were '[i]n accordance with the Rule 27 of the Olympic Charter' and that 'the work of the Organizing Committee . . . fully complies with the requirements of the Olympic Charter and the guidelines of the IOC Medical Commission'.[64] Many of these regulations were driven by the introduction and organisation of dope and gender controls in the 1960s.[65]

Dope was also of great concern at the Los Angeles Games of 1984, and several pages of the Official Report are given over to the detail of dope and gender tests. More significantly, however, is the focus on specialism/expertise in sports medicine. Although apparently Montreal had had some problems with inexperienced volunteers, Los Angeles also engaged voluntary workers and claimed not to have any difficulty finding Medical Officers who 'represent[ed] US medicine at the highest levels'.[66] Significantly, too, the Report sets down guidelines for medical provision – such as a ratio of physicians to athletes (1 per 300) and a minimum size for polyclinics and other medical facilities (400 square feet).[67] A little over 11,000 treatments were given, largely by commercial and private firms and healthcare providers.

Certain trends in Olympic Medicine should seem familiar: specialisation and the requirement that volunteers must have some specialist knowledge or expertise, and the provision of training in sports medicine and the practicalities of working at the Games for medical volunteers. There are perhaps some differences between the way services were provided in countries with strong state medical services (hence the inflated numbers of doctors and nurses in some reports) and the need to co-ordinate free services within a commercial medical culture, such as that in LA. Yet even in the UK where medical care is dominated by the NHS, the needs of private healthcare providers were important in forming sports medicine in the 1970s and 1980s. In particular the burgeoning of sports injuries clinics – both those inside and without the NHS – proved problematic to BAS(E)M and the Institute of Sports Medicine.

## Sports injuries clinics

Although the various sports injuries surveys of the 1950s and 1960s seemed to show that there was a social need for special services for the injured athlete, it was not until the 1970s that those with a vested interest in sports medicine made concerted effort to establish a chain of specialist sports injury clinics (SICs) across Britain.[68] In the first instance, these clinics were an extension of the sports injuries surveys, as their primary purpose was to record and report the cases that presented in the clinics, providing data which could be used to justify and modify future provision. But the story of the SICs is made complex by a level of 'politics' which confused and alarmed even experienced civil servants, and largely involves an enthusiastic Sports Council (now chaired by Roger Bannister), pressing for support and finance from the DHSS and the Minister for Sport, while the major sports medicine organisations were excluded, and criticised the scheme from the sidelines.[69]

What caused the division was partially a question of professional territory – which we shall address more specifically below in relation to training and education – and partially the ongoing tension between the needs of the elite and the lay body. We can pick up the story where we left off in the last chapter; Bannister had approached the Chief Medical Officer of the DHSS, George Godber, in late 1968 to discuss the treatment of sports injuries in Britain. Godber had asked for more information, and so Bannister returned in November 1971 with the results of Professor Browne's (Sports Council-funded) sports injuries survey in Newcastle.[70] Godber does not seem to have been convinced of the social need for sports clinics, but did appoint a group of advisors to make inquiries and explore the issue, the most active of whom was Dr Prophet.[71]

Dr Prophet's 'initial unease concerning Dr Bannister's proposal [were] enhanced as a result of [his] preliminary excursions into the field'; over about six months he sought opinions from doctors and surgeons working

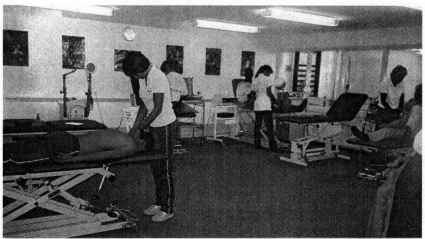

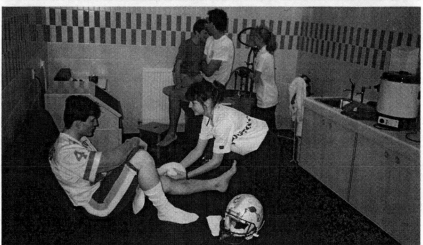

**4.** Athletes undergoing treatment at the Sports Injury Centre at the Crystal Palace National Sports Centre, *c.* 1990. The Injury Centre dates from 1976, when an ad hoc 'injuries service' was provided to athletes (many of whom were training for the Olympics in Montreal) on Tuesdays and Thursdays; Dr Frank Cramer was appointed as Medical Officer for the Crystal Palace National Sports Centre in 1977. See V Grisogono, 'The Injuries Service at the Crystal Palace' *BJSM*, 15 (1981), 39–43.

in A&E departments or in facilities recognised for their focus on sports injuries.[72] He visited Professor Browne and the surgeon Mr Petty in Newcastle, Mr Newman and Mr Sweetman (surgeons) of the Middlesex hospital, Professor Duthie at Oxford (an orthopaedic surgeon who was known to have sports injuries experience), various members of the BOA, and Dr JGP Williams and Dr Peter Sperryn.[73] The consensus opinion was that it would be a misuse of scarce NHS funds to set up SICs in the manner proposed by the Sports Council. This was an opinion held even by those who actually ran SICs, including Williams and Sperryn, whose objections will be discussed in more detail below. If sports injuries were receiving poor service – which was generally agreed – then this was reflective of a wider failure in Accident and Emergency and soft-tissue injury services, which needed a broader solution.

Here the DHSS thought it could end its involvement, but undeterred the Sports Council decided to embark on its own pilot study, which aimed to survey the need for, use, and cost of SICs.[74] Starting in February 1972 the Sports Council recruited consultants, doctors and surgeons into a scheme where they agreed to run SICs modelled on:

> a 24-hour casualty department, under a consultant orthopaedic surgeon with an interest in sports injuries, where injured sportsmen can be seen quickly . . . [with a] quick referral to a consultant in physical medicine working at the same hospital.[75]

In return for some funding, particularly for administrative costs, participants agreed to keep records on a standardised form to assess the quality and quantity of care given to patients. Importantly, the Sports Council said that '[t]he ultimate purpose of the project [was] to make out a case for improved treatment of sports injuries in particular, and soft tissue injuries in general' – already moving beyond the 'special' needs of athletes to broader issues of general health care.[76]

Initially intended to cover six to eight clinics at a cost of around £4250, the scheme expanded to twelve clinics by the end of 1973 (see Box 10).[77] Notable sports medics, and BAS(E)M members, were not represented in the scheme, in part because the eligibility rules excluded them. Sperryn was approached to take part but refused; the terms of reference meant that clinics had to be under the guidance of hospital-based consultants, which Sperryn was not, and he felt that the two orthopaedic surgeons he worked with who *would* be eligible to run a SIC would not co-operate with the scheme.[78] Dr JGP Williams was not eligible to take part because he was based at a rehabilitation centre, rather than a hospital; he told the DHSS that Bannister had pushed this pilot study through against the advice of some leaders in the field who had 'grave reservations about the validity of arguments for this type of service' and who felt that the proposed study did not have 'a sound academic basis for the proper study of the pathology and management of injuries peculiar to sport'.[79] These ongoing arguments further convinced the DHSS (and in particular Dr Prophet) that the whole of sports medicine was 'endowed with politics' which were 'diverse and deep'.[80]

Early reports from the pilot scheme were disappointing, not least because those running the clinics, some of whom had apparently no previous interest in sports medicine, were unwilling to prioritise or fast-track athletes when confronted with long waiting lists for treatment. Or, as Dr Williams framed it, many of these 'so-called' SICs were run by medical professionals (by default, surgeons) with little or no experience of sports medicine, who were not members of BAS(E)M and/or who were not recognised as part of the informal network of experts in British sports medicine.[81] As a consequence, perhaps we can infer that they did not share the opinion that the athlete was a 'privileged person' who required or deserved special treatment or consideration. Some of this critique appears to be well-founded; Dr Prophet identified just seven British 'experts' in sports injuries (with hospital or medical centre connections) in his early survey in 1972–73, and of these only two were involved in the Sports Council's Pilot Scheme. Of the original twelve Sports Council clinics, only half were still running in 1978 (see Box 10).[82]

To add to the 'politics', in October 1973 the Council of Europe passed resolution (73)27, 'On the Establishment of Sports Medicine Centres'.[83] This resolution, like their previous proclamations, linked sports medicine to health and insisted that 'sports and physical activities must not be the exclusive preserve of certain age groups and *special categories of persons* such as selected athletes [my emphasis]'.[84] It made five key recommendations, all of which required government intervention; firstly to encourage teaching, practice and research in sports medicine; secondly to ensure – particularly for Sport for All activities – that all sports organisations encourage participants to be medically screened; thirdly to include sports medicine in the curricula of sports training and physical education centres; significantly to 'encourage the establishment of sports medicine centres where the need exists and the resources are available' which, fifthly, may 'make use . . . of personnel and information' from other member States.[85]

While the Sports Council had spearheaded the dismissal of interventionalist recommendations from the Council of Europe in the 1960s, they received almost identical advice very warmly in the 1970s. Yet the effect was that the divide between the amateur and elite athletic body was made explicit, and not just within sports medicine but also in the work of the Sports Council, even the DHSS.[86] Elite athletic bodies could not be catered for in basic sports injuries clinics, and facilities for elite or professional bodies were, in a practical as much as an ideological sense, not appropriate for amateur sportsmen and women and their Saturday injuries.

The final report of the Sports Council's Pilot Study of SICs was published in 1976. As well as providing the desired epidemiological and demographic information on the percentage of injuries, the sites of injury, which sports caused the most casualties and so on, the report articulated a very strong *ideological* stance on future sports injuries provision. Of the 1636 patients:

> most were male, ordinary club or casual players, of socio-economic grade C1, employed men, and from the area around the clinics. Many were students and school-children. Only 8% were internationals and 3% professional.[87]

The possibility that international and professional players might be seeking the 'expert' service of the many sports medics who had been excluded from the study is not considered.

Of course, a concentration on the general public may have seemed to be the only way to get the DHSS's interest, but it is an ambiguous and danger-ous position for sports medicine. Although it has been broadened out into the public sphere, and is explicitly, in the Sports Council's interpretation, a 'broad, community problem', it is at the same time considerablynarrowed into a mere A&E/soft tissue and orthopaedic service (with perhaps some rehabilitation).[88] This is some distance from the holistic, multi-specialty, interdisciplinary, academically rigorous medical specialism BAS(E)M thought it should be. This model of sports medicine (or rather: of sports *injuries* medicine) is also embedded in hospitals and under the guidance of surgeons or orthopaedic consultants and not GPs or other specialists in community clinics. It is therefore unsurprising that the increasingly GP-led BAS(E)M focused on 'expertise', reaffirmed its 'special' knowledge through the body of the elite athlete, and remained sceptical of the general purpose SIC run by what many members thought of as 'non-experts'.

### Healthy sports

As the last chapter made clear, as far as sports medicine and sports science funding were concerned, the Sports Council had focused on the elite athlete and on high performance physiology. This changed in the 1970s. The SICs scheme is one example, but there are even more explicit refer-ences to a deliberate shift towards promoting sport as a health benefit, and providing medical support at all levels of sporting participation. Prompted by the Sport for All campaign, in 1971 the Sports Council admitted that 'the Research and Statistics Committee has never squarely faced the complex issue of the relationship of sport . . . to 'fitness' and health'.[89] Given that 'successive ministers' had promoted community sport as a health benefit, while others 'question the scientific justification for relating sports participation directly to 'fitness'', the Council thought it ought to start new research in this area.[90] Historically, while 'Britain has been greatly interested in establishing fitness training methods and programmes for particular sports', the Council thought in 1971 that '[w]e are happier and more at ease arguing that sport is fun . . . than arguing for increased opportunities on grounds of the community's physical health'.[91]

The Sports Council's attitude was clearly affected by changes in its organisation, and in government interest in sport in the 1970s. In 1972 the Council was reformed as an executive agency by the Conservative government, which involved absorbing several functions (and the grant-giving ability) of what remained of the Central Council of Physical Recreation, which now acts as a spokes-organisation for British sport. This almost inevitably refocused some of the Council's attention on matters traditionally of interest to the CCPR, i.e. school sports, access to leisure facilities, etc. Sports medicine became perhaps more important to the Council as Roger Bannister – a sportsman and a doctor, if not a sports doctor – became chairman, while Peter McIntosh (a key figure at the Institute of Sports Medicine) became the new chair of the Research Committee.

The reason for increased government interest in sport and leisure is complicated, and discussed elsewhere; usually what historians focus on are concerns with urban crime and deprivation, the pressure of European movements such as Sport for All, and consequent increased demand from the public and sports lobbies for increased facilities.[92] But what writers on the politics of sport and leisure management have not engaged with is the concurrently changing attitudes in public health, which were increasingly interventionalist, increasingly based on the principle of altering individual lifestyles, increasingly able to cope with complicated epidemiological problems of risk and reward and increasingly keen to use surveys and other surveillance methods to analyse complicated relationships between behaviour and disease.[93] While the Sports Council were perhaps slow to take up new trends in public health which may have their roots in the 1960s, it is clear that a significant change occurred in its attitude towards lay sport and exercise for health between 1970 and 1975.

Through the early 1970s the Sports Council continued to fund the investigation into exercise in middle-aged men; regular meetings were held to discuss fitness and health; and surveys of literature and research in other nations took place. Nonetheless, the Council was sometimes still wary of being actively involved in the promotion of exercise or sport on the grounds of health or fitness; for example, in 1973 a proposal to publish a simplified version of a 'pamphlet on exercise, fitness and health prepared by Dr Edwards at the suggestion of the Chairman [Bannister]' was rejected, because the '[Research] Committee had serious misgivings about the Sports Council publishing the shortened version. It was felt that comment on exercise systems and their value to health was more appropriate to the Department of Health and Social Security'.[94]

This position was to change in 1976; in that year the DHSS met with the Sports Council to discuss the evidence for a link between health and exercise. As a consequence the Sports Council undertook to engage in research specifically focusing on connections between longevity, health, fitness and sport – notably a large-scale literature review by Professor PH Fentem, an expert in heart disease, which ran between 1977 and 1978 (later known as the 'Fentem Report').[95] Fentem's findings were key in providing justification for a link between health and sport which was promoted by the Sports Council from 1978 onwards. BAS(E)M were not convinced of the value of Fentem's work, feeling that original research would be more productive than a literature review, which could only reveal what was already known. Their complaints led to the formation of the 'Medical Advisory Group' in 1976, a joint committee with the Sports Council, which was intended to 'assist the Sports Council on medical aspects of an exercise campaign'.[96] This joint advisory group lasted less than two years.

The Medical Advisory Group's dissolution in 1978 was caused in part by external factors. A response to the Council of Europe's Resolution on Sports Medicine was due in 1978, and in July of that year the Minister for Sport wrote to the Sports Council to ask their advice on 'certain aspects of sports medicine and science in Britain'.[97] Meanwhile, the tightening of the NHS budget had led to closure threats for some of the SICs on the Sports Council's Pilot scheme, and users wrote to both the Minister of Sport and the DHSS in protest.[98] Consequently a 'Sports Science and Medical Working Group' was appointed to make recommendations on the long-term future activity of the Sports Council in these areas. In its report, produced in 1978, it recommended that the Medical Advisory Group should disband 'with thanks for a job well done', and that the Sports Council should pay more attention to 'ethical' issues, particularly foul play and doping.[99] The Medical Advisory Group left a legacy, however; in March 1978 it had persuaded the Sports Council to 'give a new impetus to the Sport For All campaign by linking it with exercise and health'.[100]

The rest of the report produced by the Sports Science and Medical Working Group re-emphasised the distance between the elite and the lay athletic body.[101]

> The sportsman needs rapid diagnosis and accelerated treatment, to enable him to get back to sport and to some extent work. For the higher levels of competition, this need is greater and more justified ... The higher levels of competition are also more likely to benefit from the advice and services of physiologists, nutritionalists, biochemists and psychologists ... we therefore make a wide range of recommendations to improve the knowledge of the

existing hospital doctors, GP's [sic] and physiotherapists . . . and to under-pin these growing services with a limited *but* highly skilled and specialised research base. [original emphasis].[102]

Conversely, for the 'great mass of injuries incurred by Club sportsmen and users of public facilities' what was needed was better general treat-ment for soft tissue injuries, and the employment of registrars and senior physiotherapists in general hospitals (first aid facilities ought also be expanded).[103]

The elite or professional sportsman (and the gender is male throughout the report), required more than the lay exerciser. Extensive and costed rec-ommendations were made in the report to increase the money available to national teams for the training of their medical advisers, access to screen-ing, drug testing, and specialised training advice. The division between the elite and lay body was explicit. The next challenge was to formalise the process of expert recognition in sports medicine. 'Sports medicine and science', the report asserts, 'is underpinned by a very random and insecure base of knowledge and skills. There is no recognition nor career prospects to attract large numbers of good committed people'.[104] BAS(E)M was to be used as a conduit for grants for training doctors and medical auxilia-ries; £200,000 should be made available to procure two Chairs in Sports Science and Medicine, to teach not just medical undergraduates but also students on sports and physical education degree courses. This prelimi-nary report eventually became the basis for SC(79)12, the Sports Council's first formal statement of policy relating to sports medicine and science.[105]

### Sports medicine as a specialty

One of the reasons why Williams and Sperryn were not supportive of SICs when asked by Dr Prophet was that neither thought the UK had enough experts in sports medicine to establish a suitably sized pilot study. It would be unreasonable, they argued, to assess the value of a specialist service based on a survey of clinics run in the first instance by non-experts. The related discussions about specialist services and experts in the 1970s draw a clear distinction between the establishment of sports medicine as a formal medical specialty (which would involve hospital consultancies and formalised postgraduate training) and the recognition of specialists in sports medicine (i.e. institutional and social recognition of men and women with experience and expertise in treating athletes).

In the 1970s the mainstream opinion in BAS(E)M and other organisa-tions seems to have focused more on the latter, informal, definition of sports medicine. Calls for the former, more formalised recognition do not generally emerge until the late 1970s, but then much more strongly in the 1980s. As we have already seen, the Sports Council, in response to the Council of Europe's *Medical Aspects of Sport*, dismissed the idea that sports medicine should be a specialty in 1969. Less than a decade later its Sports Science and Medical Working Group argued the exact opposite position: 'the great problem [for sports medicine provision] was that sports medicine was not a recognised specialty'.[106]

The reasons why the British medical profession and individual sports medicine experts might object to the development of a formal specialism are multiple and complex, and are discussed in more detail within the broader discussion of specialisation in Chapter 6.[107] In the following sections I will focus particularly on the demands for better sports medicine education in the 1970s and 1980s. (These reforms did eventually form the backbone for claims to specialty status in the 1990s).

Discussions about, and attempts to provide, special education for sports medicine are interwoven into other disputes. For example, in 1972 the BOA came under criticism by the British print press because of the way they were managing the Olympic Team. BAS(E)M took advantage of this tide to specifically pick on the failings of the BOA in terms of sports medicine, and in turn to highlight BAS(E)M's own expertise in this area. An editorial in the *British Journal of Sports Medicine* contrasts the scientific and administrative medical demands of the international sporting scene with the apparent complacency of the BOA, who were allegedly not appointing the 'best' men for the job. The editorial suggests that the BOA should 'publi[sh] a clearly defined job description in respect of the Honorary Medical Officers and the services which they are required to provide', and goes on to 'invite the [BOA] to fill all its offices by open public competition'.[108] The implication that the BOA were appointing staff from an internal 'old-boys network' was extended to the auxiliary staff, with the suggestion that the BOA turned a blind eye to 'unqualified persons' being taken with the team as physiotherapists (the BOA promised to stop this practice in 1974).[109]

These debates about specialism and education are also reflected in the ongoing priority dispute between BAS(E)M and the Institute of Sports Medicine. The Institute was nominally the 'academic' wing of sports medicine in Britain, and therefore was an obvious candidate to organise and provide any specialist education. But training is a mechanism of authority; those who controlled the educational path of the next generation of sports medicine specialists could eventually control sports medicine, especially since specialism and education are so closely intertwined – a 'necessarily distinct training path' is and was a criterion for the recognition of medical specialism in the UK.[110] There is also an economic aspect at play here,

as by the early 1980s the demands for specialist sports medicine services were high enough to sustain dozens of private clinics. While sports
medicine may not have been lucrative, it was clearly possible to make a
living from it outside the NHS, and those doctors who wanted to do so
needed mechanisms to display their expertise to paying customers.[111]
They would presumably support any representative body which enabled,
through courses and certificates, their recognition as an 'expert' (if not a
'specialist') in sports medicine.

In 1976 the Institute of Sports Medicine, responding to the Conjoint
Board's decision to create a Diploma in Physical Rehabilitation, began to
lobby the Royal Colleges for a diploma in sports medicine.[112] The executive
of BAS(E)M, however, continued to be 'firmly opposed to this approach'.[113]
There were three reasons for this objection: firstly, sports medicine was a
'multi-disciplinary proposition' and no system of specialisation active in
the UK could adequately recognise that. Secondly (an ongoing complaint)
European models were being used as the standards for specialty, but these
standards were below even the existing informal standards in the UK,
and were entirely inappropriate as models for British specialty formation.
Thirdly, BAS(E)M 'members [were] well and truly bored . . . by the intricacies and manoeuvrings of the Institute', and these would surely only get
another outing with the inevitable struggle for control over the process of
specialisation.[114]

But *something* needed to be done. The issue of specialist training was
caught up in the debates about SICs, because specialist centres raise
questions about the need for expertise as much as the need for specialist
treatment. Calls, from BAS(E)M and individual members, for regulation,
education and recognition of experts were increasingly used as a way to
distinguish between genuine practitioners and quacks.[115] This is a classic
– almost symptomatic – feature of the development of many medical
specialisms (see Chapter 6). It was even possible to use the perceived
need for specialist education to deflect more general criticisms of sports
medicine. In 1980, in an article which was to become notorious, the orthopaedic surgeon Dr Pringle condemned sports medicine as a 'pseudospecialty' which he claimed was 'dangerous, meddlesome and wasteful'.[116]
In response, at least one sports medicine expert (Dr, later Professor, JE
Davies, an MRCP with a Diploma in Physical Medicine) turned Pringle's
argument against sports medicine in general into a specific attack on
'unqualified 'back street' sports injuries clinics'.[117] So Pringle's argument
that it was 'artificial' to group patients 'according to the origin of their
injuries' was entirely inverted to favour the creation of comprehensive,
formalised, privately provided and regularised sports medicine clinics.

There is an emphasis in Davies' article on *private* provision of sports medicine. Fairly regularly in the course of the DHSS and Sports Council's studies into SICs they had been told that private health care, particularly specialist insurance, was the best way to provide services to athletes. Davies later argued for a personal insurance-based system of sports medicine provision, an argument which provoked another controversy. In 1980 the British Association of Trauma in Sports (BATS) was formed, ostensibly by those doctors who wished to push harder than BAS(E)M for formal specialist recognition. According to some practitioners 'sports medicine [had] acquired a quite undeserved reputation among some of the medical profession as a specialty which harbours some quacks and charlatans'.[118] The presence of a doctors-only organisation might help combat this reputation.

But as well as providing this doctors-only space, what BATS also did was enter into negotiations with an insurance company, CT Bowring, to provide specialist medical insurance for athletes.[119] This led to an extraordinary accusation of corruption by Sperryn, then honorary secretary of BAS(E)M; '[f]ounder members of BATS' he claimed in his Hon. Secs. column in the *British Journal of Sports Medicine*, were 'also [a] medical advisory team to an Insurance company which has launched a sports insurance scheme'.[120] The implication was that founding BATS was essentially a self-serving activity: the organisation would decide who was and who was not a sports medicine expert, while at the same time having a financial interest in an insurance scheme which would use such experts. Sperryn withdrew these accusations, strongly rejected by BATS members, in a subsequent column, although having done so he then printed the names of four officers of BATS, followed by four medical advisers to Bowring's 'sportcare' scheme – and the lists are identical.[121] Sperryn's opinion was not isolated:

> the majority of the [Executive] Committee [of BAS(E)M] have steadfastly questioned the claims of anybody to accredit specialist expertise in sports medicine in the absence of clearer academic objectives: it has also repeatedly sought to clarify the organisational and ethical principles involved. The membership should know of the Executive Committee's difficulties which at times included the need to tape record proceedings and suspend minutes, a quite unprecedented situation in the Association's history.[122]

The insurance scheme offered by Bowring fell through, and although the BATS managed to attract perhaps up to 200 members, and ran for several years, attendance at its AGMs was sometimes less than 10% of the membership.[123] But the desire for a society which would specifically protect the needs of doctors in sports medicine was apparently strong; in 1982 a 'Registered Medical Practitioners Sub-Committee' was formed within BAS(E)M, to consider the formation of a central – possibly federal – sports medicine organisation. Such an organisation would maintain the inter-disciplinarity of sports medicine, while allowing sub-groups, in this case doctors, to have specialist organisations which would protect their own interests.[124] This is another classic indicator of specialty formation, as it is effectively a closing of ranks to protect expertise. Though obviously about broadening sports medicine, creating a federation of many bodies, it is implicit that these are to be co-ordinated by *doctors*. In this context, debates over specialty and specialism were re-cast as much narrower matters of practitioner training. So the desire for recognised authority in sports medicine, of final authority over the elite athletic and lay athletic body, distinguished not only between trained mainstream and 'fringe', but also (and perhaps most divisively) between doctors and other medical services.

In 1981 the Institute of Sports Medicine arranged with the London Hospital Medical College (affiliated with the University of London) to provide a Diploma in Sports Medicine.[125] The first course started in October 1982, it was full time (four days a week for 24 weeks) and was 'intended for medically qualified personnel and aim[ed] to provide a sound theoretical and practical training for doctors responsible for the health and care of athletes engaged in all forms of sport'.[126] The fees were fairly steep – £3200 for British and European Economic Community citizens, and £5500 for international graduates.[127] After three years the course had turned out just 19 diplomates, of whom only three were British practition-ers; the cost, the time commitment and the absence of any obvious career path (e.g. consultancy positions) in sports medicine were blamed for the low throughput of UK students.[128]

But the high number of foreign graduates had a surprising up-side for some BAS(E)M members, who used it as part of an argument for the estab-lishment of a new sports medicine institute, and associated diploma. The incoming Chairman of the Greater London Council Arts and Recreation Committee in 1984, Peter Pitt, was apparently 'very keen on what they did in Eastern Europe', with regard to recognising sports medicine as an aca-demic and clinical specialty.[129] Approaching BAS(E)M members he asked about the possibility of a GLC Chair in Sports Medicine, only to have it pointed out to him that such a person would almost certainly be a foreign graduate. Instead, between 1984 and 1986 negotiations went on between the Greater London Council and BAS(E)M to found an institute for sports medicine in London, to act as a research and educational hub for *British* sports medics.[130] On the day that the funds of the GLC were finally frozen (after a fairly aggressive move by the Thatcher government to close the Council, then under the chairmanship of Ken Livingstone) £650,000 was transferred to BAS(E)M for what became the London Sports Medicine Institute (LSMI), initially based in rooms at St Bartholomew's Hospital.[131]

The Diploma offered at the LSMI was a part-time course, and therefore much more attractive to general practitioners and experienced medical graduates already in full-time work. This Diploma could be gained over three years by attending lectures on Wednesday evenings.[132] As well as lecture rooms and a library the LSMI also had a 'physiological testing laboratory' and 'clinical examination . . . rooms'.[133] Its course considered the special needs of elite, Olympic-level, athletes, and at the same time looked at how sport could contribute to fitness, and to the health of the general population. (BAS(E)M had also introduced its own part-time course at Bisham Abbey in 1984).

## Conclusion

In 1989 the Royal Society of Apothecaries launched a Diploma in Sports Medicine. The courses at the LSMI, BAS(E)M and the London Hospital were all recognised as part of this diploma, alongside a dissertation and some other requirements. Thus a Royal College-approved formal 'educational path' was available for medical graduates interested in sports medicine. The syllabus for this diploma includes the telling phrase '[p]rescribing exercise to the unathletic'.[134] The widespread use of this sort of 'exercise as drug' metaphor begins to appear prominently in Britain in the 1970s, and is pervasive by the 1980s, especially in the language of fitness and health used by the DHSS, the Health Education Council and the Sports Council.

In 1975 Sperryn and Williams had made the argument that Sport for All necessarily meant 'Sports Injuries for All'; if the government were going to encourage the public to exercise, then there was an inbuilt responsibility to provide the services needed to make sport 'safe', not least adequate sports medicine interventions.[135] Sport for All poses very difficult biomedical questions about the value of sport and exercise for the 'normal' body; given the risk of traumatic injury, long-term chronic musculoskeletal conditions, even sudden death, *was* sport a desirable activity? In a pragmatic sense this is an economic question – at what point do the benefits of increased health due to increased fitness become outweighed by the cost of exercise facility provision and sports injuries? In the mid-1970s the government turned to sports medicine experts to answer this question. Having established that the athletic body was a strange clinical phenomenon, best understood through studies in exercise physiology and practical experience, sports medics had carved themselves a medical niche of expertise. The studies and researches which began to answer the government's (particularly the DHSS's) queries emphasised the need for regulation and control, for tailoring the sport and exercise to meet the patients' needs, and in particular for sponsoring and accrediting specialist sports medicine centres, institutes and clinics.

The increasing 'lay' participation in sports, particularly endurance sports, in the 1970s and '80s could have presented a serious challenge to the emerging professionalism of sports medicine, threatening to subsume it as mere 'fitness' in general practice, or regard its specific injuries as nothing more than mainstream soft tissue or orthopaedic injuries, to be directed to the relevant parts of general hospitals. Yet despite the increasing governmental, scientific and medical attention on lay sport, the athletic body remained clinically intact. It had been a discrete and defined clinical entity (and also a special sort of patient group) in 1970 and remained so in 1987, although – and perhaps in relation to Sport for All/the Leisure Revolution – it was increasingly being seen as abnormal as much as supernormal, and perhaps unhealthy in the long-term. The pressing question for this period was, instead, could a lay body safely take part in a specialist activity? The answer was yes, just so long as that lay body undertook a programme of adaptation – euphemistically called 'training' – which would produce enough of an athlete's body to allow safe exercise. This should not be attempted, of course, without the advice of a doctor, and ideally a sports medicine expert, who would also be the only person fully qualified to guide and assess such training. And it may be advisable (certainly in the 1980s) for any such patient to consider a specific health insurance programme to cover their new, 'special', sporting needs, for which they would be assessed and treated, again, by a sports medicine expert. Luckily, these experts were now much easier to find; not only were they often members of a professional organisation, but increasingly they had attended courses, and held diplomas or certificates.

Not all of the new developments were geared towards the lay body. In 1987 Princess Anne opened the British Olympic Association's Medical Centre at Northwick Park Hospital in Middlesex. The Centre 'provides facilities for the treatment of injuries sustained in sport, physical and physiological assessment and dietary advice to accredited competitors in all sports'.[136] Access to the Centre could only be gained via the authorisation of the relevant governing body of the sport in question, or the relevant Medical Officer. The medical staff consisted of two Members of the Royal College of Physicians, rather than orthopaedic surgeons, and a registered nurse, alongside a scientific staff of two physiologists and a laboratory technician.[137]

So, nearly twenty years after the first serious attempt to create medical centres for lay bodies, and nearly thirty years after the formation of the BOA's own Medical Committee, the Olympian finally had a specialised medical centre. The BOA Medical Centre was not without its critics, who argued that the money would be more fairly spent on more low-key interventions for mid-level athletes, or that this home counties/London centre was starving the provinces of funds. Nonetheless, it still represented the institutionalisation of an idea more than a century in the making – the clinically distinct and physiologically discrete body of the athlete; with it came the specialists, specialties and specialisms that regarded this body as their area of expert knowledge. Most importantly, however, in the last quarter of the twentieth century these experts had successfully negotiated to have their expertise applied to the body public, as well as the athletic body.

## Notes

1 For an overview of booms and busts in leisure, see: SG Jones, 'Trends in the Leisure Industry Since the Second World War' *Service Industries Journal* 6 (1986), 330–48; for a more focused account of governmental involvement in sport see JF Coghlan & IM Webb, *Sport and British Politics since 1960* (London: Falmer Press, 1990), especially Chapter 6.

2 JB King, 'Sports Medicine' *Journal of the Royal Society of Medicine* 79 (1986), 441–2. 441.

3 P McIntosh, *Sport for All Programmes Throughout the World: A Report prepared by Professor Peter McIntosh for the International Council of Sport and Physical Education for submission to UNESCO in November 1980* (ICSPE/UNESCO, 1980). Available to download: http://unesdoc.unesco.org/ulis

4 As quoted in McIntosh, *Sport for All*, p. 8.

5 RA Aronowitz, *Making Sense of Illness: Science, Society and Disease* (Cambridge: Cambridge University Press, 1998); WG Rothstein, *Public Health and the Risk Factor: A History of an Uneven Medical Revolution* (Rochester, NY: University of Rochester Press, 2003).

6 For example, see the materials relating to various health and fitness campaigns, and a White Paper on health and exercise at National Archives [hence: NA] AT60/116, AT60/117.

7 [NA]. MH166/1394. *The Sports Council, Parliament Square House, London: Proposals to establish Sports Injuries Clinics.* Letter MJ Prophet to Dr Catherine Dennis, n.d. *c.* 1971. This phrase is a neat, and almost certainly unconscious mirror of reports at the beginning of the century discussing the unwillingness of private insurance companies to cover professional athletes: 'In fact they would sooner insure a window-cleaner than a footballer.' Anon, 'En Passant: Compensation for Injuries' *Athletic News*, 1 Jul. 1907.

8 See for example: Anon, 'Rx Exercise' *Practitioner* 211 (1973), 582.

9 Anon, 'All Round Athletes: Book Review' *BMJ* 2 (1988), 1619.

10 AW Fowler, 'Sudden Death in Squash Players' *Lancet* 323 (1984), 393–4. 393; 'Editorial: Welsh Health' *Practitioner* 226 (1982), 1983.

11 Castle was the Secretary of State for the Department of Health and Social Security in Harold Wilson's cabinet (1974–76) and therefore responsible for health as well as welfare policies. 'Editorial' *BJSM* 8 (1974), 162.

12 In return, Bannister suggested that the leading promoters of sports medicine in the UK, 'certain enthusiasts' were 'way out on a limb', and that the Sports Council's interpretation of sports medicine was appropriately moderate. [NA] MH166/1394. *The Sports Council . . . Proposals to establish Sports Injuries Clinics.* Letter Owen to Mrs Reeve and Dr Prophet, 25 June 1973.

13 These were sometimes unfavourably categorised with the new 'direct-access cosmetic surgery clinics', cosmetic surgery being another specialty not formally recognised in Britain at this time: 'Editorial', *BJSM* 15 (1981), 3–4. 3. JE Davies, 'Sports Injuries and Society' *BJSM* 15 (1981), 33–4. 34.

14 S Payne, *Medicine, Sport and the Law* (Oxford: Blackwell, 1990).

15 See the cuttings in [NA] AT60/137 cited above; O Gillie, 'If You Want To Stay Fit Beware The Sporting Life' *Sunday Times*, 3 Sep. 1972.

16 Media events also provoked specific concerns, notably the collapse of President Carter in a 10km race in 1979, and the death of British boxer Johnny Owen in 1980, which confirmed some longstanding prejudices about the relative dangers of running and boxing.

17 The number of marathons run in England in the 1960s remained between six and eight; by the 1970s this had risen to around a dozen, with twenty-six in 1980, forty-seven in 1981 and 115 in 1983. [CSSH] II.M203. N McGuinness, *A Study of the Temporal and Regional Aspects of the English Marathon between 1908 and 1985, with Suggested Explanations for Trends Uncovered*, BSocial Sciences Dissertation, n.d.

18 In the early 1980s the Sports Council's Research Committee was replaced by the Fitness and Health Advisory Group, a Drug Abuse Advisory Group and a Physical Education Advisory Group. DTS Pedoe, 'Popular Marathons, Half Marathons, and Other Long Distance Runs: Recommendations for Medical Support; Recommendations of a Consensus Conference' *BMJ* 1 (1984), 1355–9.

19 Formal medical support for marathons had increased significantly in the early 1980s: BT Williams & JP Nicholl, 'Medical Arrangements in 108 Open Entry British Marathons' *Health Trends* 3 (1984), 68–70.

20 IM Sharman, 'Glycogen Loading – Advantages but Possible Disadvantages' *BJSM* 15 (1981), 114.

21 It is perhaps worth noting that the 1972 and '73 papers were sponsored by Beecham Products. DS Muckle, 'Glucose Syrup Ingestion and Team Performance in Soccer' *BJSM* 7 (1973), 340–3; LF Green & R Bagley, 'Ingestion of a Glucose Syrup Drink During Long Distance Canoeing' *BJSM* 6 (1972), 125–8; V Thomas, 'Some Effects Of Glucose Syrup Ingestion Upon Extended Sub-Maximal Sports Performance' *BJSM* 5 (1971), 212–27.

22 'The typical English Game of Football calls for greater muscular strength than any other pastime, and it is important that those who indulge in it should prepare themselves by proper diet. For this purpose there is nothing

to equal Cocoa, which in its absolutely pure form, as in CADBURY'S, contains all the elements of strength and vigour necessary to give force and firmness to the muscles and nerves, and to import staying-power to the player. Before the game, it supplies a high degree of energy; after the game, it imports a restful and comfortable feeling' Advert for Cadbury's cocoa, *Athletic News*, 24 Feb. 1896.

23  E Griffiths, 'Proceedings of the 18th World Congress of Sports Medicine: Opening Address' *BJSM* 7 (1973), 11.

24  BH Day, N Gorvindasamy, R Patnaik, 'Corticosteroid Injections in the Treatment of Tennis Elbow' *Practitioner* 22 (1978), 459–62; RL Basur, E Shepherd, GL Mouzas, 'A Cooling Method in the Treatment of Ankle Sprains' *Practitioner* 216 (1976), 708–11.

25  Anon, 'Bitter Pill for Doctors in Sports Medicine' *Times*, 4 Aug. 1972. Movement remained associated with modernity and rapid recovery, and controlled trials of rest and movement in the following years reasserted the superiority of early mobilisation. TS Little, 'Tennis Elbow – to Rest or Not to Rest' *Practitioner* 228 (1984), 457.

26  S Sheffrin, 'Medical Arrangements for the European Youth Swimming and Diving Championships' *BJSM* 3&4 (1973), 366–7.

27  CRA Clark, 'The Care of the Mountaineer' *Practitioner* 217 (1976), 235–9. 235.

28  PN Paterson-Brown, 'Poor management of unconscious rugby player watched by millions' *BMJ* 1 (1984), 1229.

29  Anon, 'How to Find a Sports Injury Clinic' *Running Magazine* 68 (1986), 46.

30  N Wilson, 'Why British sport is losing patients' *Sportsworld* 4 (1975), 9–11. 10.

31  [CSSH] SOR(WGI)14. Letter Dr Brooke to the Minister of State for Sport, 21 May 1974.

32  Ibid.

33  [NA] AT60/65. Studies and Research into Sport, Exercise and Health. Appendix B to Paper 4- Grant Application to the Sports Council, June 1977; [NA] AT60/118. Studies and Research into Sport, Exercise and Health. Newspaper cuttings relating to Loughborough jogging study. c. October 1978; [CSSH] SC(78). *Minutes of the Executive Committee.* 10 July 1978;

34  CSB Galasko *et al.*, 'University of Manchester Sports Injury Clinic' *BJSM* 16 (1982), 23–6. 23.

35  Ibid.

36  The 'Centre of Excellence' scheme in the North West listed Olympic-level sportsmen in the region – about a hundred names – excluding professional sportsmen. This was based on a list of elite athletes drawn up by the Sports Council. See the oral evidence of Professor Charles Galasko (b.1939) in LA Reynolds and EM Tansey (eds) *The Development of Sports Medicine in Twentieth-Century Britain (Transcript of a Witness Seminar)* (London: Wellcome Trust, 2009), p. 42; Galasko, 'University of Manchester SIC'.

37  MD Deveraux & SM Lachmann, 'Athletes attending a sports injury clinic – a

review' *BJSM* 17 (1983), 137-42; [NA] FD23/4515. *Medical Research and Sport.* Outline proposals for the Cambridge project, n.d.

38 E.g. MS Bourne, 'The Effect on Healing of Analgesic and Anti-inflammatory Therapy' *BJSM* 14 (1980), 26.

39 'Editorial' *BJSM* 8 (1974), 162.

40 Personal Collection of Dr Malcolm Read [Hence: MR] Letter New Allied Medical Assurance Services Limited to Malcolm Read, 19 Jan. 1984; similar definitions were used by other companies, for example: Letter Dr K Middleton, 1984 Provident Trust, to Malcolm Read, 13 Oct. 1989; Letter Christopher Darke, CMO PPP to Malcolm Read, 29 Nov. 1979.

41 [BAS(E)M]. *Minutes of the Executive Committee.* 25 Sept. 1968; Anon, 'International Federation and Sports Medicine Minutes' *Journal of Sports Medicine* 16 (1976), 1–2.

42 BAS(E)M was asked to contribute to the design and content of this new course. 'Editorial' *BJSM* 8 (1974), 67.

43 R Harland, 'Sport and Exercise Medicine – a Personal Perspective' *Lancet* 366 (2005), s53–4; various witnesses, Reynolds & Tansey, *The Development of Sports Medicine.*

44 As an example, in 1974 Salford began to offer a BSc in Human Movement Studies and Physiology which had a strong sports medicine/science component. Anon, 'Miscellaneous Notices' *BJSM* 8 (1974), 129.

45 Dr Hugh Burry, FRCP, had been in the New Zealand All Black rugby team, and was the convener of BAS(E)M's special sub-committee on 'Sudden Death in Sport'. [CSSH] SC(75) *Minutes of the Executive Committee.* 25 Feb. 1975.

46 [CSSH] SC(RS)70. *Minutes of the Research and Statistics Committee.* 17 Mar. 1970 and appendix marked SC(RS)(70)12; [NA] FD23/1289. Rehabilitation after Cardiac Disease.

47 J Rhodda, 'Research Down the Middle' *Guardian,* 24 Apr. 1970.

48 For more on heart disease and 'exercise prescriptions' see: V Heggie, 'A Century of Cardiomythology: Exercise and the Heart c1880–1980' *Social History of Medicine* (Online advance access, 2009).

49 R Owen, 'A Preliminary Evaluation of Altitude Training; Particularly as carried out by some members of the Olympic Teams of Great Britain and of other European Countries' *BJSM* 8 (1974), 9–11. 10.

50 Anon, 'Boxing Injuries: BMA Calls for Evidence' *BMJ* 1 (1983), 495.

51 'Editorial' *BJSM* 17 (1983), 74–5. 75.

52 Organising Committee of the Games of the XXth Olympiad, *The Official Report of the Organising Committee of the Games of the XXth Olympiad, Munich, 1972* (Munich: The Organising Committee of the Games of the XXth Olympiad, 1972). Vol 1, p. 374.

53 See the evidence of Dr Malcolm Read, in Reynolds & Tansey, *The Development of Sports Medicine,* pp. 41–2.

54 [BOA] 13.1 BOA HDBK. *Team Handbooks.* Official Handbook of the XXth Olympiad, Munich, 1972.

55  Ibid, Official Handbook of the XXIth Olympiad, Montreal.

56  Organising Committee of the Games of the XXIth Olympiad, *The Official Report of the Organising Committee of the Games of the XXIth Olympiad, Montreal, 1976* (Montreal: The Organising Committee of the Games of the XXIth Olympiad, 1976), p. 455.

57  Ibid., p. 457.

58  [BOA] 13.1 BOA HDBK. *Team Handbooks.* Official Handbook of the XXIIth Olympiad, Moscow, 1980.

59  Ibid., p. 6.

60  Ibid.

61  Ibid., p. 7.

62  Ibid., p. 7.

63  Organising Committee of the Games of the XXIIth Olympiad, *The Official Report of the Organising Committee of the XXIIth Olympiad, Moscow, 1980* (Moscow: The Organising Committee of the Games of the XXIIth Olympiad, 1980), p. 324.

64  V Rogozkin, 'Medical Service at the 1980 Olympic Games' *Journal of Sports Medicine and Physical Fitness* 19 (1979), 417-19, p. 417.

65  The rules did not guarantee satisfactory medical support, as evidence by the detailed condemnation of health care and hygiene at the Seoul Games in 1988: JR Axon, 'A Personal Report on the Seoul Olympic Games, 1988' *BJSM* 23 (1989), 56–7.

66  Organising Committee of the Games of the XXIIIth Olympiad, *The Official Report of the Organising Committee of the Games of the XXIIIth Olympiad, LA, 1984* (LA: The Organising Committee of the Games of the XXIIIth Olympiad, 1984). 360.

67  Ibid., p. 364.

68  JGP Williams, 'Sports Injuries – the Case for Specialised Clinics in the United Kingdom' *BJSM* 9 (1975), 22–4.

69  As one civil servant in the Department of Health and Social Security wrote in 1973: 'The politics, the suggestion of rivalry among the groups associated [with] Sport is incredible. We must proceed [with] care + caution.' [NA] MH166/1394. *The Sports Council ... Proposals to Establish Sports Injuries Clinics.* Handwritten note, possibly Dr Prophet to Dr Laylock, 20 Dec. 1973.

70  [CSSH]. SC(RS)(68)3. Note of a meeting held at the Ministry of Health on Wednesday 19THNovember 1967 at 4pm; [NA] MH166/1394. *The Sports Council ... Proposals to Establish Sports Injuries Clinics.* Notes of a meeting re. Sports Injuries, 26 Nov. 1971.

71  The membership of the advisory group is unclear, but letters on this issue are generally sent to a group including: Dr MJ Prophet, Dr Catherine Dennis, Dr Archibald and Dr Yellowlees.

72  [NA] MH166/1394. The Sports Council ... Proposals to Establish Sports Injuries Clinics. Letter Dr Prophet to Dr Dennis, n.d. c.Feb. 1972.

73  Ibid. Letter Dr Prophet to Drs Archibald and Yellowlees, 4 May 1972. For a

biography of Dr Peter Sperryn see Reynolds & Tansey, *The Development of Sports Medicine*, pp. 128–9.

74 The DHSS did not formally approve or authorise the Sports Council's project, but did generally assist it by writing to the relevant Health Authorities to ask them to support the clinics if possible. By September 1973 no participants had written back asking for extra DHSS support. [NA] MH166/1394. *The Sports Council . . .Proposals to establish sports injuries clincs*. Letter Dr Owen to Dr Prophet, 17 Sep. 1973.

75 Ibid. Letter BJ Rees to Dr Owen, 25 June 1973.

76 [CSSH] SC(IR)(73)6. Sports Injury Clinics, 7 Feb. 1973.

77 Ibid.

78 [CSSH] SC(IR) File Note by Dr Bannister Following His Recent Telephone Conversation with Dr Peter Sperryn, 18 Oct. 1972.

79 [NA] MH166/1394. The Sports Council . . . Proposals to Establish Sports Injuries Clinics. Letter Dr Williams to Dr Philips, c.1974.

80 [NA] MH166/1394. Letter Dr Prophet to Dr Yellowlees, 3 June 1974; Letter Dr Prophet to Dr Dennis, n.d. *c.* 1972.

81 [NA] MH166/1394. Letter Dr Williams to Dr Philips, c.1974.

82 [NA] MH166/1394. Letter Dr Prophet to Dr Dennis, 14 June 1972.

83 Council of Europe Committee of Members, *Resolution 73(27) On the Establishment of Sports Medicine Centres*, Adopted 25 Oct. 1973. Available on the Council of Europe website: https://wcd.coe.int

84 Ibid., p. 1.

85 Ibid., p. 2.

86 Of course, the divide had long been recognised by international bodies – see the League of Nations proclamations in the late 1930s in Chapter 3.

87 [NA] MH166/1394. *The Sports Council . . . Proposals to Establish Sports Injuries Clinics*. The Sports Council Pilot Study of Sport Injury Clinics, Dr KJ Kingsbury.

88 Ibid., 'Conclusions'.

89 [CSSH] SC(RS)(71)6. Sport and Exercise – Fitness and Health, 5 Mar. 1971.

90 Ibid.

91 Ibid.

92 B Houlihan, *The Government and Politics of Sport* (London: Routledge, 1991), Chapter 4 'The Sports Council and the Role of Government Agencies', pp. 82–114; HJ Evans, *Service to Sport: the story of the CCPR, 1937 – 1975* (London: Pelham (in association with the Sports Council), 1974).

93 V Berridge, 'Medicine and the Public: The 1962 Report of the Royal College of Physicians and the New Public Health' *Bulletin of the History of Medicine* 81 (2007), 286–311; V Berridge, *Health and Society in Britain since 1939* (Cambridge: Cambridge University Press, 1999), 85–93.

94 [CSSH] SC(IR)(73). *Minutes of the Research Committee*. 10 Apr. 1973.

95 See materials on Fentem in [NA] AT60/65. *Studies and research into sport, exercise and health; AT60/137.*

96 [CSSH] SC(78). Minutes of the Executive Committee. 13 Mar. 1978; [BAS(E) M]. Minutes of the Executive Committee. 18 Mar. 1976.

97 [NA] MH166/1394. *The Sports Council . . . Proposals to Establish Sports Injuries Clinics. Sports Science and Medicine Working Group – Summary Report*, n.d. Summer 1978

98 [NA] AT60/65. *Studies and Research into Sport, Exercise and Health.* Letter Mr Pilbeam to Mrs O'Shea, 11 May 1978; Letter Mr Butler to Mr Ellingham, Apr. 1978.

99 [NA] MH166/1394. *The Sports Council . . . Proposals to Establish Sports Injuries Clinics. Sports Science and Medicine Working Group – Summary Report*, n.d. c. Summer 1978.

100 [CSSH] SC(78). Minutes of the Executive Committee. 13 Mar. 1978.

101 The makeup of the Sports Science and Medicine Working Group is unclear; it was 'drawn up' by the General Purposes Committee of the Sports Council, implying that some members of the Group may have come from outside bodies – such as BAS(E)M which had been represented on the Medical Advisory Group.

102 [NA] MH166/1394. *The Sports Council . . . Proposals to Establish Sports Injuries Clinics. Sports Science and Medicine Working Group – Summary Report*, n.d. c. Summer 1978.

103 Ibid.

104 Ibid.

105 Although it is worth pointing out that many in sports medicine felt that the promise of this document was unfulfilled. 'The Sports Council has made token efforts to promote sports medicine – usually by encouraging experts to give freely. It studiously evades the clinical issue by allowing its generous grant for "sports science" and enormous expenditure on dope control to masquerade as "sports medicine".' P Sperryn, 'SC(79)12 – A Decade On' *BJSM* 23 (1989), 144.

106 [CSSH] SC(RS)(69)10. Medical Aspects of Sport, 19 Sep. 1969 [Section IV: Training of Specialist Doctors]: SC(78). *Minutes of the Executive Committee.* 10 July 1978.

107 See also: V Heggie, 'Specialisation Without the Hospital: The Case of British Sports Medicine' *Medical History* 54 (2010), 457–74.

108 'Editorial' *BJSM* 6 (1972), 94–5. 95.

109 [BAS(E)M] Minutes of the Executive Committee. 14 Mar. 1974.

110 [NA] MH166/1394. The Sports Council ... Proposals to Establish Sports Injuries Clinics; letter WM Hollyhock to McGregor, 9 Nov. 1971.

111 And, of course, some doctors were being paid for their work for sports clubs, professional and in some cases amateur too. Evidence of Dr Michael Hutson in Reynold & Tansey, *The Development of Sports Medicine*, p. 48.

112 [BAS(E)M] Minutes of the Executive Committee. 14 May 1976.

113 'Editorial' *BJSM* 10 (1976), 83.

114 Ibid.

115 Sperryn, 'SC(79)12'.

116 RG Pringle, 'Dangerous, meddlesome, wasteful ... Sports Medicine is a Pseudospecialty' *World Medicine*, 22 Mar. 1980.

117 Davies, 'Sports Injuries and Society', 83. See the short biography of Professor Davies in Reynolds and Tansey, *The Development of Sports Medicine*, p. 116.

118 J Jones, 'Sports Medicine and Soft Tissue Lesions' in H Berry, E Hamilton, J Goodwil (eds), *Rheumatology and Rehabilitation* (London: Routledge, 1983), 127–38. 137.

119 Evidence of Professor. Davies in Reynolds and Tansey, *Development of Sports Medicine*, pp. 53–4.

120 P Sperryn, 'Secretary's Column: Unity or Fragmentation?' *BJSM* 15 (1981), 88–9. 88.

121 P Sperryn, 'Secretary's Column: The British Association of Trauma in Sport – An Apology' *BJSM* 15 (1981), 287–9.

122 Anon, 'Report of the BAS(E)M AGM 1981' *BJSM* 15 (1981), 142. [BAS(E)M] *Minutes of the Executive Committee*. 12 Jan. 1981, 11 May 1981, 24 July 1981.

123 [BAS(E)M] Minutes of the Executive Committee. 23 June 1982.

124 [BAS(E)M] Minutes of the Registered Medical Practitioners Sub-committee. 22 Feb. 1982.

125 [BAS(E)M] Minutes of the Executive Committee. 11 May 1981.

126 Advert, *BJSM* 16 (1982), 32.

127 Adjusting to 2008 figures, comparing with the change in average earnings, these fees are significant, nearly £13,000 for home students and over £22,000 for those from overseas. Lawrence H. Officer, 'Five Ways to Compute the Relative Value of a UK Pound Amount, 1830 to Present,' MeasuringWorth, 2008. www.measuringworth.com/ukcompare/ (accessed January 2010).

128 H Fazey, 'The Injury Debate. Teaching Sports Medicine – Who Pays?' *Running* 36 (1984), 74–5, 77. 74.

129 Evidence of Tunstall Pedoe in Reynolds & Tansey, *Development of Sports Medicine*. 62–3. 62.

130 [BAS(E)M] *Minutes of the Executive Committee*. 23 Aug. 1984, 19 Feb. 1985, 12 Mar. 1985, 11 Sep. 1985, 1 Nov. 1985, *c*.18 Feb. 1986.

131 [BAS(E)M] Letter Tunstall Pedoe to 'David', *c*. 18 Feb. 1986; D Tunstall Pedoe, 'Chairman's Message' *BJSM* 20 (1986), 2.

132 H Williams, 'The London Sports Medicine Institute', *BJSM* 23 (1989), 7–8. 7.

133 Ibid.

134 FB Gibberd, 'Society of Apothecaries Diploma in Sports Medicine' *BJSM* 26 (1991), 180–2.

135 P Sperryn & JGP Williams, 'Why Sports Injuries Clinics' *BMJ* 2 (1975), 364–5.

136 Anon, 'Report on the British Olympic Medical Centre Northwick Park, Middlesex' *Physiotherapy in Sport* 10 (1987), 10–11.

137 [CSSH] II.B72. [promotional leaflet] British Olympic Medical Centre – Northwick Park Hospital & Clinical Research Centre.

---

## Box 10. Sports injuries clinics

The clinics involved in the Sports Council's pilot study are listed below in the left hand column. Those which were still running in 1978 are marked with *. In the right hand column is a list of all the 'experts' in sports medicine in Britain in 1972, according to a survey by Dr Prophet.

| Institutions | 'Experts' |
|---|---|
| * Birmingham General | |
| Brook General Hospital | Mr J Buck |
| Cuckfield Hospital, Sussex | |
| Derbyshire Royal Infirmary | |
| Guy's Hospital | Dr H Burry (but Sports Council clinic run by Dr T Gibson) |
| * Hackney Hospital | |
| * Joint Services Medical Rehab Unit, Surrey Portway Hospital, Dorset | |
| * St Charles Hospital | |
| * St James Hospital | |
| * Westminster Hospital | Dr I Curwen (initially at Queen Mary's) |
| Withington Hospital, Manchester | Dr JGP Williams (Farnham) |
| | Dr P Sperryn (Hillingdon) |
| | Mr A McDougal (Victorian Infirmary, Glasgow) |
| | Dr K Lloyd (United Cardiff Hospitals) |
| | Dr J Blonstein (Amateur Boxing Association) |

The Sports Council's list of institutions in 1978 contains those starred above plus Addenbrookes (Mr B Meggitt), The Athlete's Clinic at Middlesex Hospital (Mr Sweetham), and Bristol Royal Infirmary (Mr Stableforth).

See also:
Records created or inherited by the Department of the Environment, and of Related Bodies. National Archives. AT60/65. *Studies and Research into Sport, Exercise and Health.*
Records created or inherited by the Ministry of Health and successors. National Archives. MH 166/1394 The Sports Council, Parliament Square House, London: Proposals to Establish Sports Injuries Clinics.

# 6

# Conclusion: specialty, 1988–2005

In 1988, with the Royal College of Apothecaries' Diploma in Sports Medicine still a year away, British sports medicine did not yet have a clear path to specialty. What it did have was extraordinary momentum. An interested medical practitioner could attend one of many week-long courses run by BAS(E)M (including 'refresher' courses as well as the basic introductory week); take the part-time three-year diploma for GPs at the London Sports Medicine Institute; take the full-time one-year London Hospital Course in Sports Medicine; or they could attend a week-long sports medicine course organised by the Edinburgh Post-Graduate Board for Medicine. Such opportunities were not limited to doctors – qualified physiotherapists could also enrol on a two-year, part-time course leading to a diploma in sports physiotherapy with the Association of Chartered Physiotherapists in Sports Medicine.[1]

Between 1975 and 1992 around 1500 doctors (most of whom were GPs) took the FIMS-approved BAS(E)M courses.[2] These graduates, and those from other courses, had a vested interest in ensuring that sports medicine was a career with prospects and structure. In what was probably the last significant survey of self-identifying sports medicine practitioners before the formal recognition of sports medicine as a specialty nearly 76% of respondents were male, nearly 50% were GPs and nearly 40% already had either a diploma or postgraduate qualification in sports medicine (and presumably many more had taken shorter courses).[3] Just over 86% believed that sports medicine should be recognised as a medical specialty.[4]

Spearheading the move for specialisation was a hardcore of BAS(E)M members and active sports medics. Some of them viewed the early 1990s as years of disappointment after the educational successes of the late 1980s. In particular, the relationship between the Sports Council and BAS(E)M again became acrimonious when the former took over the London Sports Medicine Institute and reformed it as the National Sports Medicine Institute (NSMI).[5] High hopes were dashed as the Sports Council 'didn't know what to do with it', removing the BAS(E)M-friendly chairman, 'sequestering' the library and threatening the funding of the newly established Education Officer.[6] The conflicts are most pointedly told through Peter Sperryn's uncompromising editorials in the *British Journal of Sports Medicine*, which criticise the Sports Council, the government and apathetic BAS(E)M members alike.

There is a certain irony, then, that it was BAS(E)M's long-term rival, the Institute of Sports Medicine, which perhaps finally enabled sports medicine to be recognised as a medical specialty in Britain. Both an 'official' and a probably apocryphal version of this story exist; both agree that the pivotal moment was a dinner held in 1996 to celebrate the awarding of the Prince Philip Medal in Sports Medicine to Professor Archie Young. Prince Philip, The Duke of Edinburgh, had been an Honorary Fellow of the Institute of Sports Medicine since its founding in the 1960s and was invited as a guest of honour to the dinner at St James's Palace. The possibly apocryphal version of the story suggests that a cunning seating plan, placing Prince Philip next to the Chair of the Conference of Royal Medical Colleges – Dame Fiona Caldicott – ensured that royal pressure was placed on the head of the body responsible for making the final judgement about specialism.[7]

The more formal version of this story, told in the pages of the *British Journal of Sports Medicine*, suggests that at this dinner Dame Fiona 'gave an address which [had] major implications for the future of sports medicine in the British Isles. She announced the establishment of a Board of Sport and Exercise Medicine'.[8] Her announcement at the dinner itself suggests that it was not a spontaneous decision taken under royal pressure, but rather the consequence of longer-term activity. The Institute of Sports Medicine had formed a working party to draw up recommendations for the future of sports medicine the previous year, and had lobbied the Royal Colleges for specialty recognition. This working party had been taken over by the NSMI, which led to some bad feeling, and PR problems, as the NSMI 'didn't understand how medical royal colleges worked, and . . . offended them'.[9] Obviously by the 1996 dinner some of this lost ground had been recovered.

This was the beginning of what became a nearly ten-year process, resulting in the submission of an application for specialty status in 2004, finally approved by the Department of Health on 21 February 2005, and entered into the Specialist Order (the official register of specialties) in September that year. The process of specialty formation is bureaucratic; the Intercollegiate Academic Board of Sport and Exercise Medicine was formed to consider the issue in 1998, but it was not until 2003 that a working party was set up to actually fill in the application form. This was streamlined by the formalised system of creating specialisms that is now embedded in the NHS, which, as of 2001, had thirteen 'principles' for specialty recognition, including the requirement that forming a specialty was 'the best and most effective way of answering a service need, or exceptionally a national need'.[10]

This book has shown that some form of sports medicine was being practiced in Britain in the early twentieth century; BAS(E)M was formed in 1952, and yet the recognition of sports medicine as a formal specialty in the UK is a feature of the twenty-first century. It is not unreasonable for commentators to ask why it took 'so long' for specialty status to be achieved. Indeed, while sports medicine in Britain is grossly understudied, one of the few truths about it is taken to be the fact that British sports medicine has always lagged, in research, prestige, practice, funding and institutions, behind world leaders in sport and sports medicine. But just as this book has shown that sports medicine existed – in what was sometimes a world-leading form – prior to the formation of BAS(E)M, so we will conclude by reconsidering Britain's 'place in the world'. The following section will compare the story of sports medicine in Britain with that across the world.[11]

## International sports medicine

Criticisms of British sports medicine have come at least as often from within than from without; in fact, self-deprecation seems far more common than the critique of external observers. As such these stories are tools used at times of uncertainty, or when the rhetoric of Britain's failure on the world-stage is needed to generate funds and support. We see specific references to the failure of British sports medicine in response to poor international performances in the 1940s and 1950s, around the time of the founding of BAS(E)M; in relation to the manoeuvrings between BAS(E)M, BOA, the Sports Council and the Institute of Sports Medicine in the 1960s; in relation to the political conflicts between the Council and BAS(E)M in the 1970s; and in relation to the push for specialisation that began in the 1980s.

The USA has been an obvious comparator; American athletes were Britain's greatest sporting rivals at the first London Olympics in 1908 and gained an increasing number of Olympic medals through the early decades of the twentieth century before becoming one half of a sporting Cold War in the 1950s. The stereotype of the American pseudo-amateur, often a college athlete with a significant scholarship able to devote considerable time to athletic training, is an early feature of negative British accounts of foreign sportsmen (and later women). It was relatively easy to dismiss American success as the result of an ungentlemanly desire to

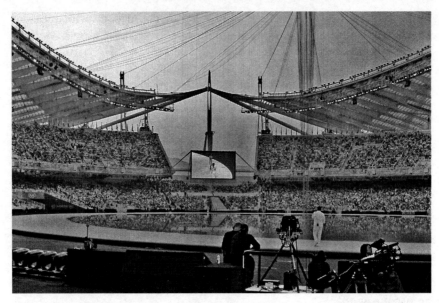

**5.** Back where it started. A packed stadium, as a large crowd watches the entertainment that formed part of the opening ceremony of the Olympic Games in Athens, 2004.

win, and an inappropriate obsession with regimented training – including advice from medical and scientific professionals.

The early history of sports medicine in the USA, as written by sports medicine professionals, usually concentrates on the work of physiologists at the turn of the century who used marathon runners as guinea pigs, and the later activity of the Harvard Fatigue Laboratory in the 1920s and 1930s.[12] Without doubt the practice of college athletics and the arrangement of international teams in the USA in the first half of the twentieth century was more ordered and competitive (and lucrative) than any comparable activity in Britain. But, when it comes to formal organisation, to professionalisation and to specialist identity, a slightly different story can be told. However informative the work of the Fatigue Laboratory and similar institutions, sports medicine in the USA could still be considered an 'undignified' activity even into the 1950s; much of the pressure to medicalise sport, or make it 'scientific', seemed to be coming from physical educators rather than doctors or physiologists.[13] Just like Britain, the USA did not get a formal organisation specifically for sports medicine (as opposed to physical fitness or physical education) until the 1950s.[14] The American College of Sports Medicine (ACSM) was founded in 1954, two years after BAS(E)M, and in the same year that the American Medical

Association formed a Committee on Injuries in Sport.[15] The ACSM did provide some educational facilities, but did 'not have a formal academic program or grant degrees'.[16]

The first specifically sports medicine-related American journal appeared in 1961, with the founding of the *Journal of Sports Medicine and Physical Fitness*, which became the ACSM's official journal in 1962.[17] And while the College offered some courses in sports medicine, even into the 1980s there was no formal postgraduate training available in the USA, '[w]ith one exception ... [t]he University of Wisconsin-Madison [which] for a period of 5 years (1967–1972), offered a postgraduate training course which was residential for eight months and granted a certificate indicating the subjects studied'.[18] Sports medicine remains only a subspecialty in the USA, with the American Board of Specialties recognising it as a sub-field (for the first time in 1992) in the overarching specialties of Emergency Medicine, Family Medicine, Internal Medicine, Orthopaedic Surgery, Paediatrics, and Physical Medicine and Rehabilitation.[19]

For other English-speaking nations, organisation and institutionalisation came even later. In Canada a joint sub-committee was formed in 1965 between the Canadian Medical Association and the Canadian Association of Health, Physical Education and Recreation, but this resulted in the founding of the Canadian Association of Sports *Science*; a medical organisation, the Canadian Academy of Sports Medicine, did not emerge until 1970.[20] On the other side of the world, the Australian Sports Medicine Federation (later: Sports Medicine Australia) was founded in 1963, producing its own journal, the *Australian Journal for Sports Medicine* for the first time in the following year; This journal later merged with the *Australian Journal of Sport Sciences* to form the *Australian Journal of Science and Medicine in Sport*, renamed in 1984 as the *Journal of Science and Medicine in Sport*. An article in this journal in 1981 describes the authors' experiences with Dr JGP Williams at Farnham Park, strongly promoting the British system as a guide for future training and educational schemes in sports medicine in Australia.[21] Whatever the failings British sports doctors saw in their own practice, it was a model for many other nations.

By the end of the twentieth century most western and northern European nations had formalised some parts of their sports medicine provision. In France the *Société Française de Médecine du Sport* had been formed as early as 1921, although sports medicine is, as of 2010, not a recognised medical specialty in that country.[22] What is sometimes cited as the first European journal of sports medicine was published by the French society from 1922 onwards – the *Revue Médecale d'éducation Physique et de Sport* – although as the title clearly demonstrates, there was considerable interest here in physical education and lay sport as much as in elite or competitive activities. By the 1980s a formal system of certification for competitive sports was introduced, making certification a legal requirement for 'the practice of competitive sport'.[23] But it was not until the 1980s that this participation certificate had to be provided by a doctor who had actually completed formal training in sports medicine.

It is notable that across Europe sports doctors engaged in many more policing activities than has been the case in Britain. Far from being 'over-cautious' about sport, medics and scientists in Britain seem to have accepted the idea that the risks of exercise and sport were parts of normal healthy manhood (and, with limits, womanhood). Elsewhere this was not always the case. The Netherlands, home to Professor Buytendijk, first president of FIMS and the reason physiological testing took place at the 1928 Amsterdam Olympics, had eleven clinics for the certification of sportsmen and women by 1930, part of a *Federatie van Bureaux voor Medische Sprotkeuring* (Federation of Bureaux for Sports Medicine Examinations).[24] In 1933 as many as 9% of those presenting for certification were declared 'unfit' to take part in any competitive sport, although it was not until 1949 that Dutch sports organisations began to systematically use the certification bureaux.

The Netherlands Association of Sports Medicine (NASM) was not founded until 1965, and for the first decade of its existence it concentrated only on the needs of the elite sporting body, moving into lay sport and sport for health in the mid-1970s (concurrent with similar changes in emphasis in Britain) when it amalgamated with the *Federatie*. Dutch training in sports medicine consisted of around forty hours of lectures, similar to those provided by BAS(E)M, from 1965 to 1975, when a longer, four-year course was introduced by the NASM. This course consisted of a year of clinical cardiology, one of clinical orthopaedic surgery, one of exercise physiology and one of practical sports medicine experience.[25] Despite this, no full-time positions in sports medicine were created in the Netherlands until 1993.

By the 1980s Sweden had a Sports Medicine Society with comparable numbers of medical members to BAS(E)M (around 700 in 1980), which ran week-long postgraduate courses, again, much like those offered by BAS(E)M.[26] Denmark had a much smaller Sports Medicine Association with fewer than 100 members, but had four sports medicine experts working permanently at University Hospital Copenhagen; meanwhile the provision of Sports Injuries Clinics in Denmark was funded, at a cost of about US$200,000 per annum, by sports organisations themselves. Finland had secured better governmental support, with the Sports Office of the Ministry of Education offering funding for sports medicine projects. The Finnish Sports Medicine Association was founded in 1939 and can make claims to being one of the oldest sports medicine organisations globally; that said, the literal translation of the Finnish means 'movement medicine', so this is another organisation with long-term, strong links to public health, with the word 'sports' avoided because in Finnish it is too closely associated only with competitive (and thus elite) sports.[27] The Finnish organisation was open only to doctors and medical students from its foundation, and ran six 'centres of research' that conducted physiological and clinical research, as well as acting as testing centres for the Finnish Olympic team. By 2000, the organisation had just 500 members, while only forty doctors had completed their training and were certified as sports medicine (or rather 'movement medicine') specialists.[28]

The USSR and Germany are two countries associated strongly with developments in sports medicine, although not always in a positive manner. It is difficult to outline the shape of sports medicine in the USSR through the twentieth century, not least because of the retrospective links made between the soviet bloc and various doping scandals. Post-1948 some government funding was allocated for physiological and biochemical research projects in sport, and '[b]y the 1970s, there were 28 Institutes of Physical Education in the USSR'; most sports historians have implied that these organisations were involved in the development of stimulants and steroids, and later blood doping and other ergogenic aids.[29] The Russian government formally acknowledged sports medicine as a discrete discipline only in 1977 (having previously referred to it as the 'medical supervision . . . of sport and physical recreation').[30]

Germany, on the other hand, has always been cited as the 'true origin' of international sports medicine. As Chapter 3 discussed, it appears to be the country where the phrase 'sports medicine' is first used, boasts the first sports medicine congress (1912), first university course (1919) and first sports medicine college (1920). That said, while the institutionalisation of what was termed 'Sports Medicine' occurred in Germany long before similar developments in Britain, it is clear that sports medicine as an *idea* was much more closely shared between the two countries. Many early German sports medicine organisations and publications were clearly linked with physical education and national fitness (particularly just prior to, and during, World War II). Practising sports doctors in the 1920s argued *against* the need for specialisation in sports medicine, because 'the physiology of sportive functioning could not be divorced from human physiology as a whole'.[31] The German athlete, even the Olympic athlete, in the 1920s was still very much in the mould of the 'normal' man, as was the case for British sportsmen and women.[32]

The post-war German Democratic Republic (GDR) formed a sports medicine organisation in 1953 (a year after BAS(E)M): the *Gesellschaft für Sportmedizin der D.D.R.* Members of this group travelled to the USSR and imported many of the practical outputs of Soviet sports medicine, including six-week 'crash' courses for GPs, and an extremely politicised focus on the performance and success of elite, international athletes. The GDR's sports medicine organisation was also pivotal in the production of *Medizin und Sport* from 1961, the first such journal published in Eastern Europe. In 1963 the provision of sports medicine was formalised, with a governmental Sports Medicine Service responsible for 'all sports medical care throughout the country'.[33]

More recently, the Turkish government formally recognised sports medicine as a specialty in 1989, instituting a three-year training scheme.[34] Despite this, into the twenty-first century there was still dissatisfaction among Turkish specialists over the limited opportunities for practice (rather than training) in Turkey. In Thailand the FIMS Diploma course was recognised by the government in the early 1970s as qualifying any MD to use the title 'Sports Doctor'; these FIMS courses were taught, in the first instance, by two sports medics from West Germany, and by Drs JGP Williams and Peter Sperryn from Britain. Like Australia, Thailand certainly saw British sports medicine as a model to follow. By 1988 Thailand had over 700 sports doctors, while all eight of its medical schools had introduced some element of sports medicine into their standard curriculum.[35]

This survey of the institutionalisation of sports medicine globally contradicts two assumptions about British sports medicine. Firstly, the allegedly sceptical and cautious British medical profession seems to have taken no part in the policing of sport so common across the continent, at least until the last quarter of the twentieth century. While in the early twentieth century some vulnerable bodies (children, women) and some extreme sports (the marathon) required medical supervision and screening, there was no suggestion – from within either sport, medicine, or government – that blanket screening should be introduced for all competitive sports. A high level of medical intervention in lay sport was flatly refused by representatives from sport and sports medicine in their responses to the Council of Europe in the 1960s.

Secondly, when we talk about the institutionalisation of sports medicine where the athletic body is a special object of clinical interest it is clear that Britain's pattern of specialty formation is roughly representative of that in most other countries considered here. It is true that other nations gained 'sports medicine' organisations earlier in the century, but these are almost exclusively those that dealt with schools sports and national fitness, an area which did not gain the same sort of medical interventionalism in Britain. Internationally, the athlete seems to have become recognised as unequivocally different in the late 1940s and 1950s, the period when many nations globally created sports medicine organisations and journals. BAS(E)M, in 1952 is therefore one of the first such organisations. More recent criticisms of sports medicine provision in Britain, particularly the idea that 2005 is a 'late' date to recognise a specialty, are undermined by the fact that few countries have formally recognised sports medicine in its own right (rather than as a sub-specialty), and most of them began to establish Chairs, Consultant posts (or equivalent) only in the 1990s and after the turn of the twenty-first century.

## Specialisation

Histories of specialisation and professionalisation have been a staple in the History of Medicine for at least two generations, and as such are, as one reviewer has put it, 'untrendy'.[36] Weisz has highlighted their tendency to teleology; while this book has explicitly laid out 'a history of' an area of medical practice which is now a specialty it should be clear that specialism was not inevitable and that sports medicine itself was not a homogenous entity over the twentieth century.[37] That said, asking questions about sports medicine *as* a specialty can still be informative and provocative. It is worth querying why sports medicine became a specialty, why in Britain it is a speciality associated with general practice, and most interestingly why, once a professional organisation was formed in 1952, for twenty-five years its members strongly denied the need for formal specialist recognition, when for the second twenty-five years of its existence so many of them appear to have thought specialisation (or at very least formal recognition and certification) was almost essential to the survival of their profession.

As Weisz has pointed out, many histories of medical specialism treat individual specialities as professions in microcosm; to a limited degree sports medicine could therefore act as a fairly useful case study in professionalisation. Through the twentieth century it gains those things usually listed as marker of a profession: first a specialist body of knowledge, then self-identity and professional unity (through organisations), then monopoly of practice (or at least the attempt to gain a monopoly) and autonomy.[38] These features map roughly onto Chapters 2, 3 and 4/5 respectively. Along the way sports medicine has gained all the trappings of a scientific or medical profession: organisations, institutions, a journal, special education and lastly state-sanctioned (specialist) recognition.

What this book has argued is that sports medicine as a discrete specialism (or micro-profession), rather than an area of expertise, could only exist when and where the athlete was considered to be a discrete clinical entity. Although the most recent work on specialisms has suggested that medical specialties emerged in the nineteenth century based on 'knowledge production and dissemination rather than as a type of skill or form of practice', such an argument does not seem to fully characterise sports medicine.[39] For the years it remained an informal specialty, practice was central. Experience, expertise and their patient's special needs were integral to the identity and self-justification of the sports medicine practitioner. Conversely the drive to make sports medicine a formal specialty had an extraordinarily complex set of motives, from professional protectionism, to jostling for power among organisations, to straight-forward financial imperatives.

There are, therefore, some unusual features of sports medicine as a specialty which shed light not only on the specific intricacies of health, sport and science, but are also reflections of distinct national themes in both sports history and the history of medicine. Sports medicine is, in Britain, an extremely non-specific specialty, which even after formal recognition still identifies itself as intrinsically multi-disciplinary.[40] This may explain its most distinctive feature – it is not a hospital-based specialism. Medical specialism in Britain, for most of the twentieth century (and indeed the nineteenth) has been a hospital-based phenomenon, and the general mechanism for specialist recognition was through consultant posts in hospitals. Sports medicine, on the other hand, was conceived as a holistic practice, including physiotherapists, coaches, and trainers, as well as doctors and surgeons.

In recent years, certainly from the late 1960s, GPs have regularly formed the single largest sub-group among the medical members of BAS(E)M. One sports medicine specialist (an orthopaedic surgeon) listed in 1986 the special training needs of sports doctors, including: pharmacology, physiology, anatomy, statistics, psychology, ENT, environmental hazards, infectious diseases, nutrition, rheumatology, gynaecology and 'the problems of the disabled'.[41] He noted the accusation that this 'wish list' 'just define[s] a general practitioner', and counters by a direct appeal to the athletic body; the argument 'is spurious. A GP's patient population is totally different'.[42] It is the patient which makes the specialism, not the scientific knowledge, biomedical discipline, or disease localisation.

Resistance to specialism is a trope in the history of medicine in Britain, closely associated with an ideal of the all-round expert, the well-educated *gentleman* doctor – often played off against the narrowly focused, incompletely educated scientist. Indeed, there are some strong resonances between the gentleman doctor, who is a good all-rounder, and the gentleman amateur, to whom sporting specialism was also anathema at least into the early twentieth century. So sports medicine shows on the one hand the development of a particularly unusual specialism – holistic, practice and patient based, and not located in the hospital. On the other hand it epitomises key themes in the history of medicine in Britain – the resistance to specialism, and the conflict between abstract laboratory science and practical clinical knowledge.

The twist in the tale is that while in the nineteenth century it was the hospital consultant who epitomised gentlemanly medicine – prioritising a holistic approach, depreciating specialism, and emphasising experience over experiment – this role was taken over in the twentieth by the general practitioner, and often, too, the sports medic. While the nineteenth century consultant was bankrolled by a list of private clients, and could work for social status, prestige and patronage within a hospital, rather than for money, the early sports doctors relied either on private incomes, or on regular jobs within the NHS (which also allowed them the flexibility to run ghost clinics and the like). It was only when, from the 1960s, some doctors sought to make a full-time career of sports medicine, or when private practitioners began to open clinics in the 1970s and 1980s, that sports medicine had to be made into a profitable practice. Specialism, certification and training seemed the only route to both profit and a protection of the professional interests of sports doctors (and, in other ways, of the interests of patients).

### 'Fitness'

At the centre of this specialist practice was a patient body – the athletic body. Towards the end of the twentieth century, sports doctors also extended their expertise to cover the public body, when it engaged in certain activities or when, crucially, it was exhorted to improve its fitness through physical exercise. Fitness is another ambiguous term; while it is often used freely, almost as if its definition is obvious, some attempts have been made by organisations in sport and medicine to come up with a definition. Some of these have been almost romantic – the 'harmony of motion' of the National Fitness Council – while others are strictly biological, comparing resting heart rates, lung capacity and so on against standardised curves and age-corrected norms.

The most important question is less often articulated – and that is 'fitness for *what?*' In the case of the athlete the answer to this question has changed over the twentieth century, while that for the lay body has remained relatively consistent. At first the question is nonsensical; 'fit and healthy' is a category which should encompass everyone, athlete and layperson. Then, perhaps, the answer became 'fit for war', or at least for the sublimated war of international sport, where athletes are avatars of their countries – representatives of the very best physical development and achievement, rather than healthy *average* normality. Finally, 'fit for purpose'; athletes who may actually live shorter lives, may be creating significant health problems through their sporting activity and may be sacrificing long-term health outcomes for short-term sporting glory.

It is the failure to answer the 'fit for what' question which has created sports medicine's biggest theoretical problems. Not least of these is the conflation of sport and health, and the athletic body and body public, which despite being constructed as clinically discrete are regularly associated both in the popular mind and in political discourse. This poses practical and social problems: sportsmen and women are used as representatives of 'health', as inspirational icons, as motivational figures. And yet the reality is that they have bodies sculpted by physical regimes and diets that no 'normal' person could emulate; they are given extraordinary levels of medical, surgical and rehabilitative care, and enhancement interventions that the lay person could not access or afford; furthermore, while they are certainly 'fit for purpose', whether that makes their model of 'fitness' an appropriate one for the rest of the population is clearly debatable. It is interesting that the only other comparable bodies which are so publically visible – those of media celebrities and fashion models – are equally unrealistic as goals, and yet are often regarded as unhealthy representations of the body, and thus unfit to be aspirational figures.

Perhaps nowhere is this coupling between the elite athletic body and the body public more obvious than at the Olympics, where bids to host the Games now absolutely require a promise of 'legacy', where the staging of the Games will provide social, sporting, economic and, crucially, health benefits to a host population. As the introduction pointed out, this is problematic in a very practical sense, as even designing infrastructure which will suit both elite and community sport is extremely challenging. And the British sports medicine community admits that there is very little evidence that major sporting events have any long-term positive impact on community health.[43] But it is also problematic in an ideological sense, where we are still trying to map the elite athletic body not only onto the body public, but also onto the 'healthy body' from which it is concurrently being disassociated (at least by doctors and by scientists). The double-think of sports medicine currently offers no answers to the problems sports and political organisations face with their division between elite and community sports.

At a time when sport, exercise and physical fitness are increasingly on the agenda of governments in the developed world, the question 'fit for *what?*' grows more important. The process by which sports medicine constructed its identity over the twentieth century – by convincingly, through expertise and experiment, answering 'for the purpose of elite sport' – has also caused it to struggle to provide a coherent answer to the question 'but is sport good for the rest of us too?'.

## Notes

1 Anon, 'Items of Interest to Members' *BJSM* 22 (1988), 170.
2 'Editorial: Sports medicine – where are the specialists?' *BJSM* 26 (1992), 75.
3 B Thompson, D MacAuley, O McNally, S O'Neill, 'Defining the sports medicine specialist in the United Kingdom: A Delphi study' *BJSM* 38 (2004), 214–17.
4 This despite the fact that around 30% of the respondents were not doctors.
5 The original GLC grant to the LSMI covered a five-year period.
6 See the evidence of Dr Dan Tunstall Pedoe: LA Reynolds and EM Tansey (eds), *The Development of Sports Medicine in Twentieth-Century Britain: Witness Seminar* (London: Wellcome, 2009), p. 65; P Sperryn, 'Editorial: New Chair – New Policies?' *BJSM* 26 (1992), 117.
7 Evidence of Dr MacLeod: Reynolds & Tansey, *Development of Sports Medicine*, p. 76.
8 D Macauley, 'Royalty, Royal Colleges, Purple Prose or Progress' *BJSM* 30 (1996), 190–1. 190.
9 See the evidence of Dr MacLeod in Reynolds and Tansey, *Development of Sports Medicine*, p. 76.
10 M Cullen & M Batt, 'Sport and exercise medicine in the United Kingdom Comes of age' *BJSM* 39 (2005), 250–1. 250.
11 For more recent developments in sports medicine education across Europe, see F Pigozzi, 'Specialisation in Sports Medicine: The State of the Sport Medicine Specialty Training Core Curriculum in the European Union', *BJSM* 43 (2009), 1085–87; E Ergen, F Pigozzi, N Bachl, HH Dickhuth, 'Sports Medicine: a European Perspective. Historical Roots, Definitions and Scope' *Journal of Sports Medicine and Physical Fitness* 46 (2006), 167–75.
12 For example, see: AJ Ryan & FL Allman Jr, *Sports Medicine* (New York; London: Academic Press, 1974), especially Chapter 2.
13 HR Collins, 'Presidential Address of the American Orthopaedic Society for Sports Medicine. Sports Medicine: Past, Present, Future' *American Journal of Sports Medicine* 17 (1989), 739–42. 740.
14 For a comprehensive study of the ACSM see J Berryman, *Out of Many, One: A History of the American College of Sports Medicine* (Champaign, Ill: Human Kinetics, 1995).
15 The Committee on Injuries was renamed the Committee on Medical Aspects of Sport and was disbanded in 1977. AJ Ryan, 'Standards for Physician Training in Sports Medicine' *Clinical Orthopaedics and Related Research* 164 (1982), 13–17. 13.
16 AJ Ryan, 'Sports Medicine Today' *Science*, 26 May 1978.
17 J Hamill, 'Biomechanics, Exercise Physiology, and the 75th Anniversary of RQES' *Research Quarterly for Exercise and Sport* 76 (2005), 53–9. 58.
18 Ryan, 'Standards in Sports Medicine', 13.
19 See the evidence of Professor Galasko in Reynolds and Tansey, *The Development of Sports Medicine*, p. 38.

20  P Safi, 'A Critical Analysis of the Development of Sports Medicine in Canada, 1955–80' *International Review for the Sociology of Sport* 42 (2007), 321–4; RJ Shephard, 'The Dimensions of Sports Medicine' *Canadian Medical Association Journal* 110 (1974), 1167–8. 1167; JAA Bullard, 'Dimensions of Sports Medicine' *Canadian Medical Association Journal* 110 (1974), 309–10.

21  PA Fricker, 'Sports Medicine Training in England' *Australian Journal of Sports Medicine* 13 (1981), 43–4.

22  F Commandré & JM Fourré, 'Sports Medicine, Preventive Medicine, and Modern Life' *Olympic Review* Part One, 188 (1983), 396–8; Part Two 190–1 (1983), 574–6. 398.

23  Ibid. Part One, 398.

24  Anon, 'History of Sports Medicine in the Netherlands' *BJSM* 23 (1989), 219–21.

25  CG Van Est, 'Sports Medicine in the Netherlands' *BJSM* 35 (2001), 5–6.

26  HE Robson, 'North West Chapter of FIMS?' *BJSM* 14 (1980), 170–8. 171.

27  O Hanninen & R Rauramaa, 'Postgraduate Degree in Sports Medicine in Finland' *BJSM* 21 (1987), 50.

28  P Kannus & J Parkkari, 'Sports and Exercise Medicine in Finland' *BJSM* 34 (2000), 239–40.

29  MI Kalinski, 'State Sponsored Research on Creatine Supplements and Blood Doping in Elite Soviet Sport' *Perspectives in Biology and Medicine* 46 (2003), 445–51.

30  J Riordan, 'Sports Medicine in the Soviet Union and German Democratic Republic' *Social Science and Medicine* 25 (1987), 19–28. 20.

31  JM Hoberman, 'The Early Development of Sports Medicine in Germany' in J Berryman and R Park (eds) *Sport and Exercise Science: Essays in the History of Sports Medicine* (Chicago: University of Illinois Press, 1992), pp. 233–81. 241.

32  This changed with the rise of the Nazi party; the superman and fascist body is a topic too large for this book, but see discussions in JA Mangan, *Shaping the Superman: Fascist Body as Political Icon – Aryan Fascism* (London: Frank Cass, 1999), in particular Chapter 4, J Hoberman, 'Primacy of Performance: Superman not Superathlete', pp. 69-85, and A Krüger, 'Breeding, Rearing and Preparing the Aryan Body: Creating Supermen the Nazi way' *International Journal of the History of Sport* 16 (1999), 42–68.

33  Riordan, 'Sports Medicine', 19.

34  H Yamen, 'Sports Medicine Training in Turkey' *BJSM* 36 (2002), 258–9.

35  C Chintanaseri, 'Sports Medicine in Thailand' *BJSM* 24 (1990), 139–42.

36  M Ramsey, 'Review: George Weisz, Divide and Conquer', *Bulletin of the History of Medicine* 81 (2007), 467–9. 468.

37  G Weisz, *Divide and Conquer: A Comparative History of Medical Specialization* (Oxford: Oxford University Press, 2005).

38  One final component, high social status, is presumably still to follow.

39  Weisz, *Divide and Conquer.* Xxi. See also, G Weisz, 'The Emergence of Medical Specialization in the Nineteenth Century' *Bulletin of the History of Medicine* 77 (2003), 536–75.

40  R Harland, 'Sport and Exercise Medicine – a Personal Perspective' *Lancet* 366 (2005), s53–4.
41  JB King, 'Sports Medicine' *Journal of the Royal Society of Medicine* 79 (1986), 441–2. 442.
42  Ibid.
43  PJ Hamlyn & ZL Hudson, '2012 Olympics: who will survive' *BJSM* 39 (2005), 882–3.

# Bibliography

*Printed sources*

Abrahams, A and AE Porritt, 'Sport and Medicine' *BMJ* 2 (1952), 98.

Abrahams, A and AE Porritt, 'Sport and Medicine' *Lancet* 260 (1952), 90.

Abrahams, A, 'Athletics and the Medical Man' *Practitioner* 86 (1911), 429–46.

Abrahams, A, 'The Scientific Side of Athletics', in EH Ryle and EE White (eds), *Athletics (The National Library of Sports and Pastimes)* (London: Eveleigh Nash, 1912), 29–40.

Abrahams, A, 'On the Physiology of Violent Exercise in Relation to the Possibility of Strain' *Lancet* 211 (1928), 429–35.

Abrahams, A, 'Athletic Training: The Olympic Standard' *Times*, 4 Aug. 1931.

Abrahams, A, 'Arterial Atony and Arterio-Sclerosis' *Lancet* 219 (1932), 480, 700.

Abrahams, A, 'Boat-Race Crews: Tests of Physical Fitness' *Times*, 31 Mar. 1933.

Abrahams, A, 'Berlin and After: The Evolution of Sport' *Times*, 24 Aug. 1936.

Abrahams, A, 'Tests for Athletic Efficiency' *Lancet* 234 (1939), 309–12.

Abrahams, A, 'Diet and Physique' *Practitioner* 155 (1945), 370–7.

Abrahams, A, 'Olympic Games; Factors in Success or Failure; The British Showing' *Times*, 13 Aug. 1948.

Abrahams, A, 'Physical Exercise – its Clinical Application' *Lancet* 257 (1951), 1133–7.

Abrahams, A, 'Amateurism in Sport' *Times*, 2 Feb. 1952.

Abrahams, A, 'Athletic Talent at Helsinki' *Times*, 31 Jul. 1952.

Abrahams, A, 'Medical Aspects of Athletics' *BMJ* 1 (1955), 1026.

Abrahams, A, *The Disabilities and Injuries of Sport* (London: Elek Books Ltd, 1961).

Abrahams, HM and A Abrahams, *Training for Athletes* (London: G Bell and Sons Ltd, 1928).

Abrahams, HM (ed.) *The Official Report of the IXth Olympiad, Amsterdam, 1928* (London: British Olympic Association, 1928).

Anderson, J, ''Turned into Taxpayers': Paraplegia, Rehabilitation and Sport at Stoke Mandeville, 1944–56, *Journal of Contemporary History* 38 (2003), 461–75.

Andrews, H and WS Alexander, *The Secret of Athletic Training* (London: Methuen & Co., 1925).

Andrews, H, Training for the Track, Field, and Road with some hints on Health and Fitness (London: Stanley Paul, 1914).

Anon, 'The Scandals of Massage: Report of the Special Commissioners of the 'British Medical Journal' *BMJ* 1 (1894), 1003–4.

Anon, 'The Medical Profession and Massage Establishments' *Lancet* 149 (1897), 538.

Anon, 'The Medical Profession and Massage Establishments' *Lancet* 152 (1898), 1073.

Anon, 'The Massage Scandals' *Lancet* 153 (1899), 1310–11.

Anon, 'Athleticism – mens sana – the Cult of Muscle' *Manchester Guardian*, 17 Jun. 1904.

Anon, 'Notes by the Way: Food Fads' *The Practitioner* 1 (1905), 852.

Anon, 'Orthodox Medical Gymnastics and Medical Massage' *Lancet* 166 (1905), 1570.

Anon, 'Massage by the Blind' *Lancet* 168 (1906), 1527–8.

Anon, 'The Olympic Games – Chances of the English Men' *Athletic News*, 16 Apr. 1906.

Anon, 'En Passant: AH Hornby's Accident' *Athletic News*, 20 May 1907.

Anon, 'En Passant: A Mishap at Liverpool' *Athletic News*, 30 Sept. 1907.

Anon, 'The Olympic Games: World's Athletes At The Stadium – Linguist, Vegetarian, Champion – the Life Story of Emil Voigt' *Athletic News*, 20 July 1908

Anon, 'Wheel World' *Athletic News*, 28 Dec. 1908.

Anon, 'En Passant: the Case of Frank Ward' *Athletic News*, 28 June 1909.

Anon, 'Notes By The Way: Races for Boys' *The Practitioner* 1 (1909), 572–3.

Anon, 'En Passant: Death of a Full Back' *Athletic News* 15 Apr. 1912.

Anon, 'Gleanings: Footballers and National Insurance' *Athletic News*, 17 June 1912.

Anon, 'En Passant: Serious accident to A Ducat' *Athletic News*, 16 Sep. 1912.

Anon, 'Une Olympiade à vol doiseau' *Revue Olympique* 80 (1912), 115–99.

Anon, 'New Mills and Newtown, Capital Racing but Poor Sport' *Athletic News*, 13 July 1914.

Anon, 'Massage Treatment – Its Value to Athletes' *Athletic News*, 20 July 1914.

Anon, 'Topics of the Track' *Athletic News*, 28 June 1915.

Anon, 'Sports Doctors' *BMJ* 211 (1928), 365–6.

Anon, 'Royal Society of Medicine: Orthopaedics – Tennis Elbow' *Lancet* 215 (1929), 1257–8.

Anon, 'Tennis Elbow' *Lancet* 215 (1930), 660.

Anon, 'Injuries and Sport, Book Review' *Lancet* 218 (1931), 638–9.

Anon, 'Injuries and Sport' *BMJ* 2 (1931), 18.

Anon, 'The Science of Exercise' *Lancet* 219 (1932), 988.

Anon 'Medical News' *BMJ* 2 (1936), 107.

Anon, 'She's Now A Man' *Daily Mirror*, 29 May 1936.

Anon, 'Olympic Games' *Time*, 10 Aug. 1936.

Anon, 'Change of Sex' *Time*, 24 Aug. 1936.

Anon, 'Medical News' *Lancet* 231 (1938), 1253.

Anon, 'Annotations: The Kidney and Exercise' *Lancet* 233 (1939), 939–40.

Anon, 'Medical Research Council Report for 1937–8' *Lancet* 239 (1939), 525.

Anon, 'Attack on Glands', *Daily Mirror* 8 Mar. 1939.

Anon, 'The Unnatural Athlete' *Lancet* 234 (1939), 211.

Anon, 'Tennis Elbow' *Practitioner* 164 (1950), 293–7.

Anon, 'A Great Runner' *BMJ* 1 (1954), 1143.

Anon, 'Sports Injuries Clinic' *Athletics Weekly* 12.38 (1958). Back cover.

Anon, 'Injuries and treatment' *Athletics Weekly* 14.48 (1960), 3.

Anon, 'The Fifth of a Series of Six Articles on the Treatment of Athletic Injuries' *Athletics Weekly* 14.9 (1960), 6–10.

Anon, 'Doping and the Use of Chemical Agents to Modify Human Performance in Sport' *BJSM* 1 (1964), 40–2.

Armstrong, JR and WE Tucker (eds) *Injury in Sport – The Physiology, Prevention and treatment of Injuries associated with Sport* (London: Staples Press, 1964).

Anon, 'Girl Athlete To Have New Sex Tests' *Daily Mirror*, 20 Sep. 1967.

Anon, 'A Brief History of the Association, with its Aims, and Possible Future Developments' *BJSM* 3 (1968), 143–8.

Anon, 'Bitter Pill for Doctors in Sports Medicine' *Times*, 4 Aug. 1972.

Anon, 'Rx Exercise' *Practitioner* 211 (1973), 582.

Anon, 'Miscellaneous Notices' *BJSM* 8 (1974), 129.

Anon, 'International Federation and Sports Medicine Minutes' *Journal of Sports Medicine* 16 (1976), 1–2.

Anon, 'AV Hill – Obituary' *BMJ* 2 (1977), 51.

Anon, 'Gland Final' *Daily Mirror*, 21 July 1978.

Anon, 'News of Members' *BJSM*, 15 (1981), 220.

Anon, 'Report of the BAS(E)M AGM 1981' *BJSM* 15 (1981), 142.

Anon, 'Boxing Injuries: BMA Calls for Evidence' *BMJ* 1 (1983), 495.

Anon, 'How to find a Sports Injury Clinic' *Running Magazine* 68 (1986), 46.

Anon, 'Report on the British Olympic Medical Centre Northwick Park, Middlesex' *Physiotherapy in Sport* 10 (1987), 10–11.

Anon, 'All Round Athletes: Book Review' *BMJ* 2 (1988), 1619.

Anon, 'Items of Interest to Members' *BJSM* 22 (1988), 170.

Anon, 'History of Sports Medicine in the Netherlands' *BJSM* 23 (1989), 219–21.

'APP', 'Neglected Sprains – Danger of Developments' *Athletic News*, 24 Apr. 1910.

'A Practicing Physician', 'Healthy Exercise, The Dangers Of Systems' *Athletic News*, 18 Apr. 1910.

Aronowitz, RA, *Making Sense of Illness: Science, Society and Disease* (Cambridge: Cambridge University Press, 1998).

Atherton, M, 'Sport in the British Deaf Community' *Sport in History* 27 (2007), 276–92.

Atkinson, P, 'Strong Minds and Weak Bodies: Sports, Gymnastics, and the Medicalization of Women's Education' *British Journal of Sports History* 2 (1985), 62–71.

Axon, JR, A Personal Report on the Seoul Olympic Games, 1988' *BJSM* 23 (1989), 56–7.

Bailey, P, *Leisure and Class in Victorian England: Rational Recreation and the Contest for Control, 1830–1885* (Toronto: University of Toronto Press, 1978).

Bailey, S, *Science in the Service of Physical Education and Sport: The Story of the International Council of Sport Science and Physical Education 1956–1996* (Chichester: John Wiley & Sons, 1996).

Bailey, S, *Athlete First: A History of the Paralympic Movement* (Chichester: John Wiley & Sons, 2008).

Baker, W, 'The Leisure Revolution in Victorian England: a Review of Recent Literature' *Journal of Sport History* 6 (1979), 76–87.

Bannister, R, 'Olympic Games in Mexico – Athletes used as guinea pigs' *Times*, 18 Apr. 1966.

Bannister, R, 'The Punishment of a Long Distance Runner' *New York Times Magazine*, 18 Sep. 1966.

Bannister, R, 'A Debt Was Paid Off In Tears: Effects of Altitude on Distance Runners in Mexico' *Sports Illustrated*, 11 Nov. 1968.

Barclay, J, *In Good Hands: The History of the Chartered Society of Physiotherapy 1894– 1994* (London: Butterworth-Heinemann, 1994).

Basur, RL, E Shepherd, and GL Mouzas, 'A Cooling Method in the Treatment of Ankle Sprains' *Practitioner* 216 (1976), 708–11.

Beamish, R and I Ritchie, 'From Chivalrous "Brothers-in-Arms" to the Eligible Athlete: Changed Principles and the IOC's Banned Substance List' *International Review for the Sociology of Sport* 39 (2004), 355–71.

Beamish, R and I Ritchie, 'From Fixed Capacities to Performance-Enhancement: The Paradigm Shift in the Science of 'Training' and the Use of Performance-Enhancing Substances' *Sport in History* 25 (2005), 412–33.

Beck, P, 'Britain and the Cold War's "Cultural Olympics": Responding to the Political Drive of Soviet Sport, 1945–58' *Contemporary British History* 19 (2005), 169–85.

Beckett, AH, 'Misuse of Drugs in Sport' *BJSM* 12 (1979), 185–194.

Bennett, WH, 'On the Use of Massage in The treatment of Recent Fractures' *Lancet* 151 (1898), 359–61.

Bennett, WH, 'The Use of Massage in Recent Fractures and Other Common Injuries' *Lancet* 155 (1900), 1569–74, 1640–3.

Berridge, V, 'Medicine and the Public: The 1962 Report of the Royal College of Physicians and the New Public Health' *Bulletin of the History of Medicine* 81 (2007), 286–311.

Berridge, V, 'Medicine, Public Health and the Media in Britain from the Nineteen-fifties to the Nineteen-seventies' *Historical Research* 82 (2009), 360–73.

Berry, H, E Hamilton, and J Goodwil (eds) *Rheumatology and Rehabilitation* (London: Routledge, 1983).

Berryman, J and R Park (eds), *Sport and Exercise Science: Essays in the History of Sports Medicine* (Chicago: University of Illinois Press, 1992).

Berryman, J, *Out of Many, One: A History of the American College of Sports Medicine* (Champaign, Ill: Human Kinetics, 1995).

Best, CH, and RC Partridge, 'Observations on Olympic Athletes' *Proceedings of the Royal Society of London, Series B* 105 (1929), 323–32.

Blonstein, J and E Clarke, 'The Medical Aspects of Amateur Boxing' *BMJ* 2 (1954), 1523–5.

Bottomley, MB, 'The Stale Athlete' *Athletics Coach* 23 (1989), 25–6.

Bourne, MS, 'The Effect on Healing of Analgesic and Anti-inflammatory Therapy' *BJSM* 14 (1980), 26.

Bramwell, C and R Ellis, 'Clinical Observations on Olympic athletes' *Arbeitsphysiologie* 1 (1928), 51–60.

British Orthopaedic Association and the Medical Commission on Accident Prevention, *Annals of the Royal College of Surgeons of England* 57 (1975), 285–95.

Buck, JE, 'Some Medical Aspects of Team Care at Home' *BJSM* 3 (1968), 121–3.

Bullard, JA, 'Dimensions of Sports Medicine' *Canadian Medical Association Journal* 110 (1974), 309–10.

Busse, EW and AJ Silverman, 'Electroencephalographic Changes in Professional Boxers' *JAMA* 120 (1952), 1522–5.

Cantor, LM and GF Matthews, *Loughborough: From College to University* (Loughborough: Loughborough University, 1977).

Carter, N, 'Metatarsals and Magic Sponges: English Football and the Development of Sports Medicine,' *Journal of Sport History* 31 (2007), 53–73.

Carter, N, 'Mixing Business with Leisure? The Football Club Doctor, Sports Medicine and the Voluntary Tradition,' *Sport in History* 29 (2009), 69–91.

Carter, N, 'The Rise and Fall of the Magic Sponge: Football Trainers and the Persistence of Popular Medicine' *Social History of Medicine* 23 (2010), 261–79.

Cathcart, EP, 'Physiological Approach to Fitness' *BMJ* 2 (1938), 273–6.

Chapman, DL, Sandow the Magnificent: Eugen Sandow and the Beginnings of Bodybuilding (Urbana: University of Illinois Press, 1994).

Chintanaseri, C, 'Sports Medicine in Thailand' *BJSM* 24 (1990), 139–42.

Clark, CRA, 'The Care of the Mountaineer' *Practitioner* 217 (1976), 235–9.

Coghlan, F and IM Webb, *Sport and British Politics since 1960* (London: Falmer Press, 1990).

Collier, W, 'The Kidney and Exercise' *Transactions of the Medical Society of London* 30 (1907), 7.

Collier, W, *School Athletics and Boys' Races* (London: J&A Churchill, 1909).

Collins, HR, 'Presidential Address of the American Orthopaedic Society for Sports Medicine. Sports Medicine: Past, Present, Future' *American Journal of Sports Medicine* 17 (1989), 739–42.

Commandré, F and JM Fourré, 'Sports Medicine, Preventive Medicine, and Modern life' *Olympic Review* Part One, 188 (1983), 396–8; Part Two 190–1 (1983), 574–6.

Cooke, MW *et al.* 'A Survey of Current Consultant Practice of Treatment of Severe Ankle Sprains in Emergency Departments in the United Kingdom' *Emergency Medicine Journal* 20 (2003), 505–7.

Cooksey, FS, 'Physical Medicine' *Practitioner* 155 (1945), 300–5.

Coote, J, 'Olympic Report Attacked' *Telegraph*, 11 Apr. 1966.

Cooter, R, 'The Meaning of Fractures: Orthopaedics and the Reform of British Hospitals in the Inter-War Period' *Medical History* 31 (1987), 306–32.

Cooter, R, Surgery and Society in Peace and War: Orthopaedics and the Organisation of Modern Medicine, 1880–1948 (London: Macmillan, 1993).

Cronin, M, 'Not Taking the Medicine: Sportsmen and Doctors in Late Nineteenth-Century Britain' *Journal of Sport History* 34 (2007), 401–13.

Cullen, M and M Batt, 'Sport and Exercise Medicine in the United Kingdom Comes of Age' *BJSM* 39 (2005), 250–1.

Cunningham, H, *Leisure in the Industrial Revolution* (London: Croom Helm, 1980).

Daniels, J, 'Altitude and Athletic Training and Performance' *American Journal of Sports Medicine* 7 (1979), 371–3.

Davies, JE, 'Sports Injuries and Society' *BJSM* 15 (1981), 33–4.

Davis, LR and LC Delano, 'Fixing the Boundaries of Physical Gender: Side Effects of Anti-Drug Campaigns on Athletics' *Sociology of Sport Journal* 9 (1992), 1–19.

Day, BH, N Gorvindasamy, and R Patnaik, 'Corticosteroid Injections in the Treatment of Tennis Elbow' *Practitioner* 22 (1978), 459–62.

De Merode, A, 'The Development, Objectives and Activities of the IOC Medical Commission' in A Drix, HG Knuttgen and K Tittel (eds) *The Olympic Book of Sports Medicine: Vol I of the Encyclopaedia of Sports Medicine* (Oxford: IOC+FIMS, 1988), pp. 3–6.

Deveraux, MD and SM Lachmann, 'Athletes Attending a Sports Injury Clinic – a Review' *BJSM* 17 (1983), 137–42.

De Wachter, F, 'The Symbolism of the Healthy Body: A Philosophical Analysis of the Sportive Imagery of Health' *Journal of the Philosophy of Sport* xi (1985), 56–62.

Dickinson, BD *et al.*, 'Gender Verification of Female Olympic Athletes' *Medicine and Science in Sports and Exercise* 34 (2002), 1539–42.

Dimeo, P, A History of Drug Use in Sport 1876–1976 (London: Routledge, 2007).

Drix, A, HG Knuttgen, and K Tittel (eds) *The Olympic Book of Sports Medicine: vol 1 of the Encyclopaedia of Sports Medicine* (Oxford: IOC+the FIMS, 1988).

Duncan, KS, *The Oxford Pocket Book of Athletic Training* (Oxford: Oxford University Press, 1948).

'Editorial' *BJSM* 1 (1964), 42.

'Editorial' *BJSM* 6 (1972), 94–5.

'Editorial' *BJSM* 8 (1974), 162.

'Editorial' *BJSM* 8 (1974), 67.

'Editorial' *BJSM* 10 (1976), 83.

'Editorial' *BJSM* 15 (1981), 3–4.

'Editorial' *BJSM* 17 (1983), 74–5.

'Editorial: Sports Medicine – Where are the Specialists?' *BJSM* 26 (1992), 75.

'Editorial: Welsh Health' *Practitioner* 226 (1982), 1983.

Elsas, LJ, RP Hayes, and K Muralidharan, 'Gender Verification At The Centennial Olympic Games' *The Journal of the Medical Association of Georgia* 86 (1997), 50–4.

Ergen, E, F Pigozzi, N Bachl, and HH Dickhuth, 'Sports medicine: a European perspective. Historical roots, definitions and scope' *Journal of Sports Medicine and Physical Fitness* 46 (2006), 167–75.

Farmer, *et al.*, 'Letter: Boys' Races' *Times*, 8 Feb. 1909.

Fazey, H, 'The Injury Debate. Teaching Sports Medicine – Who Pays?' *Running* 36 (1984), 74–5, 77.

Featherstone, DF, 'Medicine and Sport' *Practitioner* 170 (1953), 299–302.

Featherstone, DF, *Sports Injuries Manual for Trainers and Coaches* (London: Nicholas Kaye, 1954).

Ferris, EA, 'Anabolic Steroids and Sport' in J Berryman and R Park (eds), *Sport and Exercise Science: Essays in the History of Sports Medicine* (Chicago: University of Illinois Press, 1992), pp. 319–50.

Fletcher, S, Women First: The Female Tradition in English Physical Education, 1880–1980 (London: Athlone Press, 1984).

Fletcher, S, 'The making and breaking of a female tradition: women's physical education in England 1880–1980' *International Journal of the History of Sport* 2 (1985), 29–39.

Fowler, AW, 'Sudden Death in Squash Players' *Lancet* 323 (1984), 393–4. 393.

Fricker, PA, 'Sports Medicine Training in England' *Australian Journal of Sports Medicine* 13 (1981), 43–4.

Galasko, CSB *et al.* 'University of Manchester Sports Injury Clinic' *BJSM* 16 (1982), 23–6.

Gardener, KD, 'Athletic nephritis: pseudo and real' *Annals of Internal Medicine* 75 (1971), 966.

Garnham, N, 'Both Praying and Playing: "Muscular Christianity" and the YMCA in North-east County Durham' *Journal of Social History* 35 (2001), 397–407.

Genel, M and A Ljungvist, 'Gender Verification of Female Athletes' *Lancet* 366 (2005), s41.

Gerrard, DF, 'The Lord Porritt – Obituary' *BJSM* 28 (1994), 77–8.

Gibberd, FB, 'Society of Apothecaries Diploma in Sports Medicine' *British Journal of Sports Medicine* 26 (1991): 180–2.

Gillie, O, 'If You Want To Stay Fit Beware The Sporting Life' *Sunday Times*, 3 Sep. 1972.

Golinski, J, *Making Natural Knowledge: Constructivism and the History of Science* (Chicago; London: University of Chicago Press, 2005).

Goodbody, J, 'Ready, Steady, Grow: Athletes turn to Viagra', *The Sunday Times*, 22 June 2008.

Graham, JW, 'Professional Boxing and the Doctor' *BMJ* 1 (1955), 219–21.

Green, LF and R Bagley, 'Ingestion of a glucose syrup drink during long distance canoeing' *BJSM* 6 (1972), 125–8.

Griffin, FWW, *Scientific Basis of Physical Education* (London: Humphrey Milford, Oxford University Press, 1937).

Griffiths, E, 'Proceedings of the 18th World Congress of Sports Medicine: Opening Address' *BJSM* 7 (1973), 11.

Grisogono, V, 'The Injuries Service at the Crystal Palace' *BJSM*, 15 (1981), 39–43.

Guttman, L, 'Significance of Sport in Rehabilitation of Spinal Paraplegics and Tetraplegics' *JAMA* 236 (1976), 195–7.

Haley, B, *The Healthy Body and Victorian Culture* (Harvard: Harvard University Press, 1977).

Hall, DE (ed.) *Muscular Christianity: Embodying the Victorian Age* (Cambridge: Cambridge University Press, 1998).

Hamill, J, 'Biomechanics, Exercise Physiology, and the 75th Anniversary of RQES' *Research Quarterly for Exercise and Sport* 76 (2005), 53–9.

Hamilton, D, *The Monkey Gland Affair* (London: Chatto & Windus, 1986).

Hamlyn, PJ and ZL Hudson, '2012 Olympics: Who Will Survive' *BJSM* 39 (2005), 882–3.

Hanninen, O and R Rauramaa, 'Postgraduate Degree in Sports Medicine in Finland' *BJSM* 21 (1987), 50.

Hargreaves, J, *Sporting Females: Critical Issues in the History and Sociology of Women's Sports* (London: Routledge, 1994).

Harland, R, 'Sport and Exercise Medicine – a Personal Perspective' *Lancet* 366 (2005), s53–4.

Hay, E, 'Femininity Tests at the Olympic Games' *Olympic Review*, 76, 77 (1974), 119–23.

Hay, E, 'The Stella Walsh Case' *Olympic Review* 162 (1981), 221–2.

Heald, CB, Injuries and Sport. A General Guide for the Practitioner (Oxford: Oxford University Press, 1931).

Heald, CB, 'Physical Exercise and Sport as Preventives of Disease' *Lancet* 223 (1934), 413–16.

Heggie, V, 'Lies, Damn Lies and Manchester's Recruiting Statistics: Degeneration as an "Urban Legend" in Victorian and Edwardian Britain' *Journal of the History of Medicine and Allied Sciences*, 63 (2008), 178–216.

Heggie, V, "Only the British Appear to be Making a Fuss'; the Science of Success and the Myth of Amateurism at the Mexico Olympiad, 1968' *Sport In History* 28 (2008), 213–35.

Heggie, V, 'Men in Women's Sport', in M Atkinson (ed.) *Battleground: Sport* (Greenwood Press, 2008) Vol I, pp. 278–84.

Heggie, V, 'A Century of Cardiomythology: Exercise and the Heart c1880–1980' *Social History of Medicine* 23 (2010), 280–98.

Heggie, V, 'Specialisation Without the Hospital: The Case of British sports medicine' *Medical History* (forthcoming, 2010).

Heggie, V, 'Volunteers for Science: Medicine, Health and the Modern Olympic Games' in V. Nutton (ed.) *Sport, Medicine and Immortality* (British Museum, forthcoming).

Heiss, F, 'Sportmedizin im Wandel der Zeiten – 50 Jahre internationaler Sportärzteverband (the FIMS)' [Sports medicine through history: 50 years of the International Assciation of Sports Physicians (the FIMS)] *Deutsche Zeitschrift für Sportmedizin* 7 (1978).

Hill, AV, *Living Machinery* (London: G Bell and Sons Ltd, 1927).

Hill, AV, Muscular Movement in Man: The Factors Governing Speed and Recovery from Fatigue (New York; London: McGraw Hill, 1927).

Hilton, J, *On Rest and Pain* (London: JG Bell & Sons, 1877).

Hoberman, J, Mortal Engines: The Science of Performance and the Dehumanization of Sport (New Jersey: Blackburn Press, 1992).

Hoberman, JM, 'The Early Development of Sports Medicine in Germany' in J Berryman and R Park (eds), *Sport and Exercise Science: Essays in the History of Sports Medicine* (Chicago: University of Illinois Press, 1992), pp. 233–81.

Hoberman, JM, *Testosterone Dreams. Rejuvenation, Aphrodisia, Doping* (Berkeley; LA; London: University of California Press, 2005).

Holst, O, 'Letter: Massage and Movement in Sprains and Dislocations' *Lancet* 160 (1902), 1424–5.

Holt, R, *Sport and the British* (Oxford: Clarendon, 1990).

Holt, R and T Mason, *Sport in Britain, 1945–2000* (Oxford: Blackwell, 2000).

Houlihan, B, *The Government and Politics of Sport* (London: Routledge, 1991).

Houlihan, B, *Dying to Win: Doping in Sport and the Development of Anti-doping Policy* (Strasbourg: Council of Europe, 1999).

Howe, P David, *Sport, Professionalism and Pain: Ethnographies of Injury And Risk* (London: Routledge, 2004).

Howell, JD, '"Soldier's Heart": The Redefinition of Heart Disease and Specialty Formation in Early Twentieth-Century Great Britain' *Medical History* 5 (1985), 34–52.

Husson, FC, 'Lucas Championnere on Massage and Mobilisation in the Treatment of Fractures' *Annals of Surgery* 11 (1889), 359–64.

Jarvis, WD, *A Medical Handbook for Athletic and Football Club Trainers* (London: Faber and Faber, 1955).

Johnson, RE, 'Applied Physiology' *Annual Review of Physiology* 8 (1946), 535–8.

Jokl, E, *The Medical Aspects of Boxing* (Pretoria: JL Van Schaik Ltd, 1941).

Jokl, E, 'Professor AV Hill, a Personal Tribute' *Journal of Sports Medicine and Physical Fitness* 20 (1980), 465–8.

Jones, J, 'Sports Medicine and Soft Tissue Lesions' in H Berry, E Hamilton, and J Goodwill (eds), *Rheumatology and Rehabilitation* (London: Routledge, 1983), pp. 127–38.

Jones, SG, 'Trends in the Leisure Industry Since the Second World War' *Service Industries Journal* 6 (1986), 330–48.

Jones, SG, 'State Intervention in Sport and Leisure in Britain Between the Wars' *Journal of Contemporary History* 22 (1987), 163–182.

Jordanova, L, 'The Social Construction of Medical Knowledge', *Social History of Medicine* 8 (1995), 361–81.

Kalinski, MI, 'State Sponsored Research on Creatine Supplements and Blood Doping in Elite Soviet Sport' *Perspectives in Biology and Medicine* 46 (2003), 445–51.

Kannus, P and J Parkkari, 'Sports and Exercise Medicine in Finland' *BJSM* 34 (2000), 239–40.

Kayser, B, A Mauron, and A Miah, 'Viewpoint: Legalisation of Performance-enhancing Drugs' *Lancet* 366 (2005), s21.

Ker Lindsay, J, 'Medical Miscellany – Injuries to the Ankle Joint' *Athletic News*, 14 Oct. 1907.

Ker Lindsay, J, 'Medical Miscellany – Sprains of the Knee Joint ' *Athletic News*, 21 Oct. 1907.

Ker Lindsay, J, 'Medical Miscellany – Does Exercise Shorten Life?' *Athletic News*, 3 Feb. 1908.

Ker Lindsay, J, 'Medical Miscellany – Use and abuse of tobacco' *Athletic News*, 10 Feb. 1908.

Ker Lindsay, J, 'Medical Miscellany – Stages of Massage' *Athletic News*, 24 Feb. 1908.

Ker Lindsay, J, 'Medical Miscellany' *Athletic News*, 16 Nov. 1908.

Khosla, T, 'Unfairness of Certain Events in the Olympic Games' *BMJ* 2 (1968), 111–13.

King, JB, 'Sports Medicine' *Journal of the Royal Society of Medicine* 79 (1986), 441–2.

Knight, SS, *Fitness and Injury in Sport* (London: Skeffington, 1952).

Krüger, A, 'Breeding, Rearing and Preparing the Aryan Body: Creating Supermen the Nazi Way' *International Journal of the History of Sport* 16 (1999), 42–68.

La Cava, G, 'Sports Medicine' *Lancet* 276 (1960), 1144.

La Cava, G, 'Editorial: Sports Medicine in Modern Times, A Short Historical Survey', *The Journal of Sports Medicine and Physical Fitness* 3 (1973), 155–8.

Lace, MV, *Massage and Medical Gymnastics* (London: J&A Churchill Ltd, 1945).

Landsborough Thomson, A, *Half a Century of Medical Research* (London: HMSO, 1975).

Larette, CH, 'How to Get Fit and Keep So' in 'Sprinter' (ed.) *The Athletic News Handbook on Training for Athletes and Cyclists* (London: Athletic News *c.* 1902).

Lawrence, C, 'Moderns and Ancients: the 'New Cardiology' in Britain 1880–1930' *Medical History* 5 (1985), 1–33.

Lawrence, J, 'A Goalkeeper's Life Story' *Athletic News*, 30 May 1921.

Lee, HB, 'Letter to the Editor: Marathons' *Athletics Weekly* 9.33 (1955), 15, 17.

Little, TS, 'Tennis elbow – to rest or not to rest' *Practitioner* 228 (1984), 457.

Lovelock, JE, 'Physiotherapy and the Athlete' *Practitioner* 158 (1947), 226–32.

Lovelock, JE, 'Physiological and Medical Principles of Training' *Practitioner* 160 (1948), 221–9.

Lucas, CJP, *The Olympic Games 1904* (St Louis: Woodward & Tiernan, 1905).

Lucas-Championère, J, *Traitement des fractures par le massage et la mobilisation* [The treatment of fractures using massage and movement] (Paris, 1885).

Lupton, D, *The Imperative of Health: Public Health and the Regulated Body* (London: Sage, 1995).

Lynch, S, 'When Men were Men . . . and so were the Women' *Guardian*, 7 Aug. 2004.

Macauley, D, 'Royalty, Royal Colleges, Purple Prose or Progress' *BJSM* 30 (1996), 190–1.

Macdonald, R, 'Crystal Palace National Sports Centre – London, UK' *BJSM* 24 (1990), 10–12.

Mallon, B, and I Buchanan, *The 1908 Olympic Games: Results for All Competitors in*

*All events, with commentary* (North Carolina; London: McFarland and Company, 2000).

Mangan, JA, *Athleticism in the Victorian and Edwardian Public School* (Cambridge: Cambridge University Press, 1981).

Mangan, JA, "Muscular, Militaristic and Manly': the British middle-class hero as moral messenger' *International Journal of the History of Sport* 13 (1996), 28–47.

Mangan, JA, Shaping the Superman: Fascist Body as Political Icon – Aryan Fascism (London: Frank Cass, 1999).

Mangan, JA and RJ Park, (eds) From 'Fair Sex' to Feminism: Sport and the Socialization of Women in the Industrial and Post-Industrial Eras (London: Routledge, 1987).

Manning, L, 'The Last Word; I Am Sorry About Mexico's Height' *Daily Mail*, 19 Apr. 1966.

Marlin, T, 'Treatment of "Tennis Elbow" with Some Observations on Joint Manipulation' *Lancet* 215 (1930), 509–11.

Maron, MB and SM Horvath, 'The Marathon: A History and Review of the Literature' *Medicine and Science in Sports* 10 (1978), 137–50.

Massengale, JD and RA Swanson (eds), *The History of Exercise and Sport Science* (Champaign, Il: Human Kinetics, 1997).

McCrone, KE, 'Play up! Play UP! And Play the Game! Sport at the Late Victorian Girls' Public School' *Journal of British Studies* 23 (1984), 106–34.

McIntosh, P, *Sport in Society* (London: CA Watts & Co Ltd, 1964).

McIntosh, P, *Physical Education in England since 1800* (London: G Bell, 1968).

McIntosh, P, *Sport for All Programmes Throughout the World: a Report prepared by Professor Peter McIntosh for the International Council of Sport and Physical Education for submission to UNESCO in November 1980* (ICSPE/UNESCO, 1980).

McMillan, GEJ, 'Letters to the Editor: First Aid' *Athletics Weekly* 11.4 (1957), 4–5.

McNab, T, P Lovesey, and A Huxtable, *The UK Literature of Track and Field* (London: British Library, 2001).

Mennell, JB, 'The Treatment of Recent Injury by Mobilisation and Massage' *Lancet* 181 (1913), 316–17.

Mewett, P, 'Sports Training, Science and Class among British Amateur Athletes in The Mid To Late Nineteenth Century' in J Northcote (ed.) *Sociology for a Mobile World: Conference Proceedings of The Australian Sociological Association 2006 Conference* (Australia: The Sociological Association of Australia, 2006), pp. 1–10.

Miah, A, 'From anti-doping to a "performance policy" sport technology, being human, and doing ethics' *European Journal of Sport Science* 5 (2005), 51–7.

Miles, E, *Restaurant Recipes* (London: Eustace Miles, 1906).

Miles, Stanley, 'Medical Criteria in the Selection of Athletes' *Proceedings of the Royal Society of Medicine* 62 (1969), 921–4.

Milledge, J, 'Obituaries: Griffith Pugh' *Independent*, 27 Jan. 1995.

Milspaugh, JA, 'Boxing and Parkinsonism' *Practitioner* 2 (1948), 513.

Moon, GP, A New Dawn Rising; An Empirical and Social Study Concerning the

Emergence and Development of English Women's Athletics until 1960, PhD, Roehampton Institute, 1997.

Mostofi, SB (ed.) *Who's Who in Orthopedics* (London: Springer, 2004).

Muckle, DS, 'Glucose syrup Ingestion and Team Performance in Soccer' *BJSM* 7 (1973), 340–3.

Mussabini, SA, *The Complete Athletic Coach* (Methuen & Co. Ltd: London, 1913).

Mussabini, SA, Track and Field Athletics: A Guide to Correct Training (Foulsham: London, 1924).

Nannestad, I, 'John Allison and his Football hospital' *Soccer History* 9 (Autumn 2004), 42–3.

Newman, PH, JPS Thomson, JM Barnes, and TCM Moore, 'A Clinic for Athletic Injuries' *Proceedings of the Royal Society of Medicine* 62 (1969), 939–41.

Nicholls, D and J Cheek, 'The Society of Trained Masseuses and the Massage Scandals of 1894' *Social Science and Medicine* 62 (2006), 236–48.

Northcote, J, (ed.) *Sociology for a mobile world: Conference proceedings of The Australian Sociological Association 2006 Conference* (Australia: The Sociological Association of Australia, 2006).

Owen, R, 'Letters to the Editor: Medical Facilities' *Athletics Weekly* 11.7 (1957), 5–6.

Owen, R, 'A Preliminary Evaluation of Altitude Training; Particularly as Carried out by Some Members of the Olympic Teams of Great Britain and of other European Countries' *BJSM* 8 (1974), 9–11.

Park, RJ, 'Athletes and Their Training in Britain and America' in J Berryman and R Park (eds) *Sport and Exercise Science: Essays in the History of Sports Medicine* (Chicago: University of Illinois Press, 1992), pp. 57–107.

Park, RJ, 'High-Protein Diets, "Damaged Hearts", and Rowing Men: Antecedents of Modern Sports Medicine and Exercise Science, 1867–1928' *Exercise and Sports Science Reviews* 25 (1997), 137–69.

Park, RJ, 'Cells or Soaring? Historical Reflections on "Visions" of the Body, Athletics, and Modern Olympism' *Olympika: The International Journal of Olympic Studies* ix (2000), 1–24.

Park, RJ, '"Mended or Ended?": Football Injuries and the British and American Medical Press, 1870–1910' *The International Journal of the History of Sport* 18 (2001), 110–33.

Paterson-Brown, PN, 'Poor management of unconscious rugby player watched by millions' *BMJ* 1 (1984), 1229.

Payne, S, *Medicine, Sport and the Law* (Oxford: Blackwell, 1990).

Pedoe, DTS, 'Popular Marathons, Half Marathons, and Other Long Distance Runs: Recommendations for Medical Support; Recommendations of a Consensus Conference' *BMJ* 1 (1984), 1355–9.

Pedoe, DTS, 'Obituary: Dr John GP Williams' *BJSM* 29 (1995), 220–2.

Pepper, WGS, AT Fripp, and WE Tanner, 'Injuries to the Professional Association Footballer' *Practitioner* 164 (1950), 298–305.

Pick, D, *Faces of Degeneration: A European Disorder c1848–1918* (Cambridge: Cambridge University Press, 1989).

Pigozzi, F, 'Specialisation in Sports Medicine: The State of the Sport Medicine

Specialty Training Core Curriculum in the European Union', *British Journal of Sports Medicine,* 43 (2009), 1085–87.

Plesch, J, 'Arterial Atony and Arterio-Sclerosis' *Lancet* 219 (1932), 385–91, 641–2.

Porritt, AE, 'Introduction' *Physical Education* 55 (1963), xii.

Pringle, RG, 'Dangerous, Meddlesome, Wasteful ... Sports Medicine is a Pseudospecialty' *World Medicine,* 22 Mar. 1980.

Rabinbach, A, *The Human Motor: Energy, Fatigue and the Origins of Modernity* (California: University of California Press, 1992).

Ramsey, M, 'Review: George Weisz, Divide and Conquer', *Bulletin of the History of Medicine* 81 (2007), 467–9.

Randal Roberts, M, 'A Footballers' Hospital' *The Windsor Magazine* (March 1899), 511–16.

Reynolds, L and EM Tansey, *The Development of Sports Medicine in Twentieth-Century Britain* (Transcript of a Witness Seminar) (London: Wellcome Trust, 2009).

Rhodda, J, 'Research Down the Middle' *Guardian,* 24 Apr. 1970.

Riordan, J, 'Sports Medicine in the Soviet Union and German Democratic Republic' *Social Science and Medicine* 25 (1987), 19–28.

Ritchie, IR, 'Sex Tested, Gender Verified: Controlling Female Sexuality in the Age of Containment' *Sports History Review* 34 (2003), 80–93.

Robson, HE, 'North West Chapter of FIMS?' *BJSM* 14 (1980), 170–8.

Robson, HE, 'Obituary: Rex Salisbury Woods' *BJSM,* 20 (1986), 187.

Robson, HE, 'Obituary: Professor La Cava' *BJSM* 23 (1989), 198.

Rogozkin, V, 'Medical Service at the 1980 Olympic Games' *Journal of Sports Medicine and Physical Fitness* 19 (1979), 417–19.

Rolleston, H, (ed.) *The British Encyclopaedia of Medical Practice – Volume II* (London: Butterworth, 1936).

Romer, F, 'Sports Injuries' *Practitioner,* 1 (1923), 99–112.

Rothstein, WG, Public Health and the Risk Factor: A History of an Uneven Medical Revolution (Rochester, NY: University of Rochester Press, 2003).

Ryan, AJ, *Medical Care of the Athlete* (London; New York; Toronto: McGraw-Hill, 1963).

Ryan, AJ, 'Medical Aspects of Sports' *JAMA* 194 (1965), 173–5.

Ryan, AJ, 'Sports Medicine Today' *Science,* 26 May 1978.

Ryan, AJ, 'Standards for Physician Training in Sports Medicine' *Clinical Orthopaedics and Related Research* **164** (1982), 13–17.

Ryan, AJ and FL Allman Jr, *Sports Medicine* (New York; London: Academic Press, 1974).

Ryle, EH and EE White (eds), *Athletics (The National Library of Sports and Pastimes)* (London: Eveleigh Nash, 1912).

Safi, P, 'A Critical Analysis of the Development of Sports Medicine in Canada, 1955–80' *International Review for the Sociology of Sport* 42 (2007), 321–4.

Schmidt, FA and EH Miles, *The Training of the Body for Games, Athletics, Gymnastics and Other Forms of Exercise and for Health, Growth and*

*Development* (New York; London: S. Sonnenschein & Company / EP Dutton & Co, 1901).

Scruton, J, *Stoke Mandeville – Road to the Paralympics* (Aylesbury: Peterhouse, 1998).

Séguillon, D, 'The Origins and Consequences of the First World Games for the Deaf: Paris, 1924' *International Journal of the History of Sport* 19 (2002), 119–32.

Sharman, IM, 'Glycogen Loading – Advantages but Possible Disadvantages' *BJSM* 15 (1981), 114.

Sheard, KG, '"Brutal and Degrading": The Medical Profession and Boxing, 1838–1984' *International Journal of the History of Sport* 15 (1998), 74–102.

Sheffrin, S,, 'Medical Arrangements for the European Youth Swimming and Diving Championships' *BJSM* 3,4 (1973), 366–7.

Shephard, RJ, 'The Dimensions of Sports Medicine' *Canadian Medical Association Journal* 110 (1974), 1167–8.

'Sir Adolphe Abrahams' *Times*, 12 Dec. 1967.

Skillen, F, '"A Sound System of Physical Training": The Development of Girls' Physical Education in Interwar Scotland' *History of Education* 38 (2009), 403–18.

Smith, A and D Porter (eds), *Amateurs and Professionals in Post-war British Sport* (London: Frank Cass, 2000).

Smodlaka, VN, 'Sports Medicine in the World Today' *JAMA* 205 (1968), 138–9.

'Special Edition: Amateurism in Britain: For the Love of the Game?', *Sport in History*, 26 (2006).

Sperryn, P, 'The Lord Porrit – Obituary' *BJSM* 28 (1994), 78.

Sperryn, P, and Williams, JGP, 'Why Sports Injuries Clinics' *BMJ* 2 (1975), 364–5.

Sperryn, P, 'Secretary's Column: The British Association of Trauma in Sport – An Apology' *BJSM* 15 (1981), 287–9.

Sperryn, P, 'Secretary's Column: Unity or Fragmentation?' *BJSM* 15 (1981), 88–9.

Sperryn, P, 'SC(79)12 – A Decade On' *BJSM* 23 (1989), 144.

Sperryn, P, 'Editorial: New Chair – New Policies?' *BJSM* 26 (1992), 117.

'Sprinter'(ed.) *The Athletic News handbook on Training for Athletes and Cyclists* (London: Athletic News *c.* 1902).

'Strephon', 'Topics of the Track' *Athletic News*, 20 May 1913.

'Strephon', 'Topics of the Track' *Athletic News*, 1 June 1914.

Sturdy, S and R Cooter, 'Science, Scientific Management, and the Transformation of Medicine in Britain, c.1870–1950' *History of Science* 36 (1998), 421–66.

Swanston, C and R Passmore, 'Medical Services in the Small Factory' *Practitioner* 162 (1949), 405–13.

Terry, D, 'An Athletic Coach Ahead of his Time' *British Society of Sports History Newsletter* 11 (Spring 2000), 34–8.

Thines, G and R Zayan, 'FJJ Buytendijk's Contribution to Animal Behaviour: Animal Psychology or Ethology?' *Acta Biotheoretica* XXIV (1975), 86–99.

Thom, W, *Pedestrianism, or, An Account of the performances of celebrated Pedestrians during the Last and Present Century* (Aberdeen: D Chalmers & Co, 1812).

Thomas, V, 'Some effects of glucose syrup ingestion upon extended sub-maximal sports performance' *BJSM* 5 (1971), 212–227.

Thompson, B, D MacAuley, O McNally, and S O'Neill, 'Defining the sports medicine specialist in the United Kingdom: A Delphi study' *BJSM* 38 (2004), 214–17.

Thompson, J, 'John Thompson's Sportfolios – Why They Go On With Glands' *Daily Mirror*, 16 Sept. 1938.

Thorndike, A, *Athletic Injuries* (Philadelphia: Lea & Febiger, 1938).

Tittel, K and HG Knuttgen, 'The Development, Objectives and Activities of the International Federation of Sports Medicine (the FIMS)' in A Drix, HG Knuttgen, K Tittel (eds), *The Olympic Book of Sports Medicine: Vol 1 of the Encyclopaedia of Sports Medicine* (Oxford: IOC+the FIMS, 1988), pp. 7–12.

Todd, T, 'Anabolic Steroids and Sport' in J Berryman and R Park (eds), *Sport and Exercise Science: Essays in the History of Sports Medicine* (Chicago: University of Illinois Press, 1992), pp. 319–50.

Toon, E and J Golden, '"Live Clean, Think Clean, and Don't go to Burlesque Shows": Charles Atlas as Health Advisor' *Journal of the History of Medicine and Allied Sciences* 57 (2002), 39–60.

'Towards National Health', *The Listener*, 7 Apr. 1937, 655.

Tucker, WE, 'Athletic Injuries' in H Rolleston (ed.), *The British Encyclopaedia of Medical Practice – Volume II* (London, Butterworth, 1936), pp. 225–38.

Tucker, WE, 'Cricketing Injuries' *Practitioner* 162 (1949), 496–501.

Tucker, WE, 'Fitness and Training' in JR Armstrong and WE Tucker (eds), *Injury in Sport – The Physiology, Prevention and Treatment of Injuries Associated with Sport* (London: Staples Press, 1964), pp. 82–93.

Van Est, CG, 'Sports medicine in the Netherlands' *BJSM* 35 (2001), 5–6.

Van Hilvoorde, I, R Vos, and G de Wert, 'Flopping, Klapping and Gene Doping: Dichotomies Between "Natural" and "Artificial" in Elite Sport' *Social Studies of Science* 37 (2007), 173–200.

Vertinsky, P, *The Eternally Wounded Woman: Doctors, Women and Exercise in the Late Nineteenth Century* (Manchester: Manchester University Press, 1990).

Vertinsky, P, 'Old Age, Gender and Physical Activity: The Biomedicalization of Aging,' *Journal of Sport History* 18 (1991), 64–80.

Vertinsky, P, 'The Social Construction of the Gendered Body: Exercise and the Exercise of Power,' *International Journal of the History of Sport* 11 (1994), 147–71.

Vertinsky, P, 'Body History for Sport Historians: The Case of Gender and Race', in K Walmesley (ed.), *Method and Methodology in Sport and Cultural History* (Iowa: Brown & Benchmark Publications, 1995), pp. 50–62.

Vertinsky, P, 'Making and Marking Gender: The Medicalization of the Body from One Century's End to Another,' *Culture, Sport and Society* 2 (1999), 1–24.

Vertinsky, P, 'Commentary: What is Sports Medicine?' *Journal of Sport History* 34 (2007), 402–5.

Wackwitz, L, 'Verifying the Myth: Olympic Sex Testing and the Category "Woman", *Women's Studies International Forum* 26 (2003), 553–60.

Waddington, I, 'The Development of Sports Medicine' *Sociology of Sport Journal* 13 (1996), 176–96.

Waddington, I and A Smith, *An Introduction to Drugs in Sport, Addicted to Winning?* (London: Routledge, 2nd edn, 2008).

Walmesley, K (ed.), *Method and Methodology in Sport and Cultural History* (Iowa: Brown & Benchmark Publications, 1995).

Warren, R, 'The Fate of Damaged Joints: A Study of Cases of Injury, Principally Fractures, Involving Joints Treated in the Massage Department of the London Hospital' *Lancet* 174 (1909), 219–22.

Webster, FAM, *The Science of Athletics* (London: Nicholas Kaye, 1936).

Webster, FAM and JA Heys, *Athletic Training For Men And Boys: A Comprehensive System of Training Tables for All Events* (London: Shaw, 1933).

Weisz, G, 'The Emergence of Medical Specialization in the Nineteenth Century' *Bulletin of the History of Medicine* 77 (2003), 536–75.

Weisz, G, *Divide and Conquer: A Comparative History of Medical Specialization* (Oxford: Oxford University Press, 2005).

Welshman, J, 'Physical Education and the School Medical Service in England and Wales, 1907–1939' *Social History of Medicine* 9 (1996), 31–48.

Welshman, J, 'Only Connect: The History of Sport, Medicine and Society' *International Journal of the History of Sport* 15 (1998), 1–21.

Welshman, J, 'Physical Culture and Sport in Schools in England and Wales, 1900–40' *International Journal of the History of Sport* 15 (1998), 54–75.

West, JB, *High Life: A History of High-Altitude Physiology and Medicine* (Oxford: Oxford University Press, 1998).

West, S, 'Heart Strain, with Some Remarks on Training and Other Allied Cardiac Conditions' *Practitioner* 2 (1911), 137–46.

Whorton, JC, '"Athlete's Heart": The Medical Debate Over Athleticism, 1870–1920' *Journal of Sport History* 9 (1982), 30–52.

Wickets, DF, 'Can Sex in Humans Be Changed' *Physical Culture*, Jan. 1937.

Wickstead, JH, *The Growth of a Profession, Being the History of the Chartered Society of Physiotherapy, 1894–1945* (London: Edward Arnold & Co, 1948).

Williams, BT and JP Nicholl, 'Medical Arrangements in 108 Open Entry British marathons' *Health Trends* 3 (1984), 68–70.

Williams, H, 'The London Sports Medicine Institute', *BJSM* 23 (1989), 7–8.

Williams, JGP, 'Injuries and Treatment' *Athletics Weekly* 14.50 (1960), 7.

Williams, JGP, *Sports Medicine* (London: Edward Arnold, 1962).

Williams, JGP, 'Sports Injuries – the Case for Specialised Clinics in the United Kingdom' *BJSM* 9 (1975), 22–4.

Wilson, N, 'Why British Sport is Losing Patients' *Sportsworld* 4 (1975), 9–11.

Winterstein, CE, 'Head Injuries Attributable to Boxing' *Lancet* 230 (1937), 719–20.

Woodard, C, *Sports Injuries: Prevention and Active Treatment* (London: Max Parrish, 1954).

Woods, RS, 'Physical Medicine' *Practitioner* 2 (1943), 263–70.

Woods, RS, 'Beating the Clock: Evolution in the treatment of Sports Injuries' *Practitioner* 203 (1969), 329–36.

Wrynn, A, 'The Human Factor: Science, Medicine and the International Olympic Committee, 1900–70' *Sport in Society* 2 (2004), 211–31.

Wrynn, A, '"A Debt Was Paid off in Tears": Science, IOC Politics and the Debate about High Altitude in the 1968 Mexico City Olympics' *International Journal of the History of Sport* 23 (2006), 1152–72.

Yamen, H, 'Sports Medicine Training in Turkey' *BJSM* 36 (2002), 258–9.

Zöch, C, V Fialka-Moser, and M Quittan, 'Rehabilitation of Ligamentous Ankle Injuries: A Review of Recent Studies' *BJSM* 37 (2003), 291–5.

Zweiniger-Bargielowska, I, 'Building a British Superman: Physical Culture in Interwar Britain' *Journal of Contemporary History* 41 (2006), 595–610.

### Government reports and resolutions

Council of Europe Committee of Members, Resolution 73(27) On the Establishment of Sports Medicine Centres, Adopted 25 Oct. 1973.

House of Commons Committee of Public Accounts, Preparations for the London 2012 Olympic and Paralympic Games (Fiftieth Report of Session 2007–8) (London: HMSO, 2008).

Wolfenden Committee on Sport, *Sport and the Community* (London: CCPR, 1960–61).

### Websites

www.la84foundation.org/5va/reports_frmst.htm (accessed August 2009).

All the Official Olympic Reports from 1896 to 2004 are available as PDFs from the LA84 Foundation. Specifically referred to in the text are:

Amsterdam Olympic Committee, *The Official Report of the IXth Olympiad, Amsterdam, 1928* (Amsterdam: Olympic Committee of the Amsterdam Olympic Games, 1928)

Antwerp Organising Committee, *Olympic Games Antwerp 1920* (Belgium Olympic Committee, 1957).

Berlin Olympic Committee, *The Official Report of the XIth Olympiad, Berlin* (Berlin: Olympic Committee of the Berlin Olympic Games, 1936).

British Olympic Council, *The Fourth Olympiad: London 1908* (London: British Olympic Council, 1908).

LA Olympic Committee, *The Games of the Xth Olympiad, Los Angeles 1932, Official Report* (Los Angeles: Olympic Committee of the Los Angeles Olympic Games, 1932).

London Olympic Committee, *The Official Report of the Organising Committee for the XIV Olympiad* (London: The Organising Committee for the XIV Olympiad, 1948).

Lucas, CJP, *The Olympic Games 1904* (St Louis: Woodward & Tiernan, 1905).

Melbourne Olympic Committee, *The Official Report of the Organising Committee for the Games of the XVI Olympiad Melbourne 1956* (Melbourne: Organising Committee of the Melbourne Olympiad, 1958).

Mexico Organising Committee, *Official Report of the Organising Committee of the Games of the XIX Olympiad Mexico, 1968, Vol 2* (Mexico: The Organising Committee of the Games of the XIX Olympiad, 1968).

Netherlands Olympic Committee, *The Ninth Olympiad – Official Report* (Netherlands: Netherlands Olympic Committee, 1928).

Organising Committee of the Games of the XXIIIth Olympiad, *The Official Report of the Organising Committee of the Games of the XXIIIth Olympiad, LA, 1984* (Los Angeles: The Organising Committee of the Games of the XXIIIth Olympiad, 1984).

Organising Committee of the Games of the XXIIth Olympiad, *The Official Report of the Organising Committee of the XXIIth Olympiad, Moscow, 1980* (Moscow: The Organising Committee of the Games of the XXIIth Olympiad, 1980).

Organising Committee of the Games of the XXIth Olympiad, *The Official Report of the Organising Committee of the Games of the XXIth Olympiad, Montreal, 1976* (Montreal: The Organising Committee of the Games of the XXIth Olympiad, 1976.

Organising Committee of the Games of the XXth Olympiad, *The Official Report of the Organising Committee of the Games of the XXth Olympiad, Munich, 1972* (Munich: The Organising Committee of the Games of the XXth Olympiad, 1972).

Paris Organising Committee, *VIIIme Olympiade Paris 1924* (Paris: French Olympic Committee, 1924).

*Rapports – Exposition Universelle International de 1900 á Paris* [Including the Official Report of the Olympic Games] (Paris: Ministére Du Commerce, De L'Industrie des Postes et des Télégraphes, 1900).

Rome Organising Committee, The Official Report of the Organising Committee for the Games of the XVII Olympiad Rome 1960, Vol I (Rome: Organising Committee of the Rome Olympiad, 1960).

Stockholm Organising Committee, *The Olympic Games of Stockholm 1912* (Stockholm: Swedish Olympic Committee/Wahlstrom & Widstrand, 1912).

Tokyo Organising Committee, The Official Report of the Games of the XVIII Olympiad Tokyo 1964, Vol I (Tokyo: Kyodo Printing Co. Ltd, 1964).


www.measuringworth.com
Online calculators which allow various calculations of the 'value' of money, or 'cost' of items in the past (accessed December 2009).


www.wada-ama.org/rtecontent/document/QA_List_OR.pdf
Discussion by the World Anti-Doping Agency of the possible status of Viagra in future games (accessed August 2009).


https://wcd.coe.int
Search page for Council of Europe documents (accessed August 2009).


http://unesdoc.unesco.org/ulis
Search page for UNESCO documents (accessed August 2009).

## Archives

### Archives of the British Association of Sport and Exercise Medicine

The research in this book has been conducted on personal photocopies of items which have subsequently been deposited in the Wellcome Trust Library, and can be found under the general catalogue reference: SA/BSM: *Collection, British Association of Sport and Exercise Medicine*

Annual General Meetings, 1953–2000

Minutes of the Executive Committee, 1953–2000

Minutes of the Registered Medical Practitioners Sub-committee, 1982

Misc. Papers, 1953–1990

Secretary's Reports, 1982–

### John Rylands University Library of Manchester

Special Collections

ARC 4/6 Log Books 1906–8 [Agecroft Rowing Club]

Manchester Medical Collection

MMC/9/6/15/4. *Massage School*

### Centre for Sports Science and History, Birmingham University

Materials in the CSSH, previously called the National Centre for Athletics Literature, have been re-catalogued since I started research for this book. Catalogue references given here refer to the old system and may no longer be in use.

*Archives of the Amateur Athletics Association*

AAA/3/7/2, Scrapbook of the 1908 Olympics

XXV.M2 Medical Statistics on 13 Men

XXV.M2 A Abrahams, The Limit of Athletic Ability

XXV.A7 A Abrahams, The 4th Crookes Lecture, Athletic Training Past and Present,

*Archives of the Sports Council*

SC(RSC) & SC(RS) Minutes of the Research and Statistics Committee, 1965–72

SC(RS) Minutes of the Research Committee, 1973–

SC Minutes of the Executive Committee, 1965–

Misc. Papers SC(IR)

Misc. Papers SC(RS)

Appendix G. Sports Council Press Statement, 1965

M.1(G)SC9. Fitness Study Group

SC(70)6. Report on the Medical Aspects of Boxing

SOR(WGI)14 Letter Dr Brooke to the Minister of State for Sport

*Other materials*

ER188/17/4 Collection of Documents Relating to the European Public Health Committee's Report on the Medical Aspects of Sport (pub. October 1967)

II.A696 Sprinter, 'Hints on Diet' in 'Sprinter' (ed.), *The Athletic News handbook on Training for Athletes and Cyclists* (c. 1902)

II.B72 British Olympic Medical Centre – Northwick Park Hospital and Clinical Research Centre

II.M203 N McGuinness, A Study of the Temporal and Regional Aspects of the English Marathon between 1908 and 1985, with suggested explanations for trends uncovered

*National Archives, Kew*

AT60 Department of the Environment and predecessors: Sports Policy, Registered Files (SARD and SPORT Series)

– /65 Studies and Research into Sport, Exercise and Health

– /116 Studies and Research into Sport, Exercise and Health; includes Draft White Paper – on Prevention and Health

– /117 Studies and Research into Sport, Exercise and Health

– /118 Studies and Research into Sport, Exercise and Health

– /137 Studies and research into sport, exercise and health

CAB124 Offices of the Minister of Reconstruction, Lord President of the Council and Minister for Science: Records

– /1646 Medical Research: Sport

ED113 National Fitness Council: Minutes, Papers and Reports

– /49 Sub-Committees of the National Advisory Council for Physical Training and Recreation; Minutes of Meetings

– /63 Voluntary Organisations

FD1 Medical Research Committee and Medical Research Council: Files

– /2474 League of Nations

FD23 Medical Research Council: Registered Files, Scientific Matters (S Series)

– /89 PHYSIOLOGY

– /1289 CORONARY THROMBOSIS

– /4515 PHYSIOLOGY

MH166 Ministry of Health and Department of Health and Social Security: Hospital Construction, Registered Files

– /1394. The *Sports Council . . . Proposals to Establish Sports Injuries Clinics*

### Archives of the British Olympic Association

Held at the BOA headquarters, 1 Wandsworth Plain, London SW18 1EH

Materials relating to the 1948 London Olympiad (Minute book)

– 1948 Games (Organizing committee) Medical Committee 1946–8

13.1 BOA HDBK *Team Handbooks* (1928–64)

34.2 MED INJUR Materials on Sports Medicine

34.23 MED INJUR Materials on Sports Medicine

Materials relating to the Altitude Problem (Box folder)

### University College London NHS Foundation Trust Archives

Minutes of the Board of Governors (Middlesex Hospital), 1946–8

Personal Collection of Dr Malcolm Read

I would like to thank Dr Read for allowing me access to his personal collection of materials related to his work in sports medicine from the 1970s.

# Index

Note: page numbers in italic refer to illustrations, while underlined references refer to Boxes.

Abrahams
    Adolphe 35–7, <u>62</u>, 65, 76–89 *passim*, 104, 118
    Harold 35, 50
alcohol 25, 52, <u>63</u>
    *see also*: drugs in sport
Allison, John 33, <u>61</u>
altitude
    controversy about Olympics held at 10, 117–23 *passim*, 131
    training at 156
Amateur Athletics Association 100n.120, 110
amateurism
    definition and ideology 8–12, 38
    science and 16, 19, 28, 121–3
American College of Sports Medicine 186–7
Association Football 11–12, 33, 69–70
    hormone 'gland' use in 81–2
    medical criticisms of 37–8
Association Internationale Medico-Sportive 73
    *see also*: Fédération Internationale de Médicine Sportive
Athlete's Heart 29, 82
    *see also*: cardiology; sports injuries/diseases

athletic body
    definition of 7, 15–19, 105, 106–9, 117–18
    normality of 27–9, 52–3
    special needs of 67, 79–82, 90, 109, 120, 131–2, 166–7
Australian Sports Medicine Federation 187

Bannister, Sir Roger 117, 122–5 *passim*, 160–2
boxing
    medicine and 11–12, 84, 110, 118, 127–9, 156
British Association of Sport and (Exercise) Medicine
    educational activities 155, 171–2
    founding 91–2
    membership of 120, 147
    relationship with ISM 130–1, 168–9
British Association of Trauma in Sport 170
British Journal of Sports Medicine 120, 150, 184
    Editorials 168–70
British Olympic Association 34, 104, 119, 156, 168, 173–4
    altitude research project 121–3
    handbooks for athletes 115–16

British Olympic Association (*cont.*)
Medical Centre at Northwick Park
Hospital 173–4
Buytendijk, Professor FJJ 73

cardiology 79–80
*see also*: Athlete's Heart
Central Council of Physical Recreation
87–8, <u>103</u>, 165
Commonwealth Games 108
Council of Europe
Medical Aspects of Sport report
126–7
resolution (73) 27 163, 166
cycling 34, 36, 78, 112

Department of Health and Social
Security 164–72 *passim*
disability 84–6
Paralympics 85
dope *see* drugs in sport
drugs in sport 6–8
testing for 110–14
use at Olympic Games 51–2
*see also*: specific drug names

Empire Games *see* Commonwealth
Games
Everest, Mount 106, <u>143</u>, 152
exercise
potential risks of 16, 29, 65, 73, 83,
149–51, 172–3
therapeutic intervention, as a 43–51
*passim*, 156–7, 166–7

Fédération Internationale de
Médicine Sportive 73–4, <u>142</u>
female athletes 87
*see also*: sex testing
first aid 25, 110, 152
*see also:* Olympic Games
fitness 28, 87–8, 90, 164–6, 193–4
national 39–40, 65–7, 72–3,
146
National Fitness Council 67, 71

food
athletes' diets 8, 32, 42–3, 71, 80–1,
150
rationing 86
vegetarianism 39–42 *passim*, 49
football *see* Association Football; rugby
football
Footballers' Hospital 46, *27*, <u>61</u>

gender tests *see* sex testing
general practitioners 127, 172
role in sports medicine 113, 147,
164, 183, 191–3
Greater London Council 124, 171–2
gymnastics 35, 43–51 *passim*, 90,
119
*see also*: massage; physiotherapy

Harvard Fatigue Laboratory 186
Hill, Professor AV 65, 73, 76–8 *passim*,
80, <u>101</u>
hormones 81–2
*see also*: drugs in sport; sex
testing

Institute of Sports Medicine 112–13,
153–4, 168–9, 171, 184
insurance
personal 154–5, 170
team  116
International Olympic Committee 1,
36, 73–4, 117, 157–9 *passim*
Medical Committee of 111–12
*see also*: drugs in sport; Olympic
Games; sex testing

laboratories 71, 109, 153, 172
Crystal Palace, at 106–7, 124, *161*
Olympic Games, at the 117
Lazaro, Francesco 35–6
League of Nations 72, 90
leisure revolution 4, 18, 145–6
Lindsay, Dr J Ker 45–9 *passim*
London Sports Medicine Institute
171–2

Loughborough College/University *69*, 89, 109, 119, 155

marathon *see* running
massage 43–51
Medical Research Committee/ Council 71, 86–7, 106–8, 122, 124, 156
Miles, Eustace 42
military 34, 45–7, 50, 66–7, 76, 84–5, 88
    research relevant to sports medicine 17, 86–7
moderation 36–43
Mussabini, Sam 50–1

National Fitness Council *see* fitness

Olympic Games 33–6, 72–9, 114–18, 157–60
    Amsterdam (1928) 75, 79
    Athens (1896) 33–4
    Berlin (1936) 76, 110–11
    Helsinki (1952) 77–8
    London (1908) 34–5, 51–2
    London (1948) 76–7, 84
    London (2012) 4, 194
    Los Angeles (1932) *13*, 75–6, 78
    Los Angeles (1984) 159–60
    Melbourne (1956) 114–15
    Mexico City (1968) 117, 121–4
    Montreal (1976) *13*, 157–8
    Moscow (1980) 158–9
    Munich (1972) 157
    Paris (1900) 33–4, 49–50
    Paris (1924) *62*, *102*
    Rome (1960) 108, 115–16
    St Louis (1904) 51–2
    Stockholm (1912) 35–6
    Tokyo (1964) 116
Oxo 32

physical education, 31, 39–42, 52, 90–1, 118–19, 126–7
physiology 28–9, 40, 65, 71–82 *passim*, 86–9, 108–9, 129, 153

physiotherapy 46–50, 70, 183
    *see also*: gymnastics; massage
Porritt, Sir Arthur *102*, 130
public health 4, 14, 19, 126, 145–7, 165
    at Olympic Games 75, 114–16
Pugh, Dr LGCE 122–4, <u>143</u>

qualifications
    Diploma in Physical Medicine 88, 113
    Diploma in Sports Medicine 155, 167, 171–2, 183
    *see also*: massage

Royal College of Physicians 88, 128, 156
Royal Society of Apothecaries 172
rugby football 31–2, 39
running
    cross-country 40–1
    marathons 51–2, 82, 110
    *see also*: Olympic Games

screening
    before participation in sport 18, 52
    Olympics, at 51–2
    unpopularity of in Britain 190
sex testing 1, 110–14
soccer *see* Association Football
specialisation 191–3
specialty status 82–3, 160–4, 167–72, 183–5
    outside the UK 185–90
Sperryn, Dr Peter 162, 170, 184, 190
Sport for All 145–7, 163–6, 172–3
Sports Council 14, 107–8, 122–31 *passim*, 149–56, 160–4, 168
    reorganisation as an executive body 165–6
sports injuries/diseases
    athlete's foot 75, 78, 115
    fractures 43–51
    sprains and strains 43–51, 88, 110

sports injuries/diseases (*cont.*)
　surveys of 108–9, 125, 129, <u>142</u>,
　　163–4
sports injury/medicine clinics 160–4,
　166
　British Olympic Association's 173
　Middlesex Hospital's 100n.120, 120
　university-based 153–4
sports science 15, 80, 84, 129, 153,
　166–8
staleness 37, <u>63</u>
Stoke Mandeville Hospital 85–6
　*see also*: disability
strychnine 16, 37, 52, <u>63</u>

training 5, 16, 25–6, 37–43, 48–9, 70–3
　*passim*, 120–4
　altitude 156
　manuals and guides 14, 28, 30–2

vegetarian *see* food
Viagra 7
Voigt, Emil 49
volunteers
　amateurism, and 3, 10–11, 127
　sports medicine, in 25, 31, 70–2,
　　151–2
　'Volunteers for Science' <u>142</u>

Walasiewiczówna, Stanislawa *see*
　Walsh, Stella
Walsh, Stella 1, 110–11
　*see also*: sex testing
war *see* military; food
Webster, FAM 69, 71
Weston, Mark (née Mary) 111
Williams, Dr JGP 108–9, <u>144</u>, 162–3,
　187, 190
Woods, Dr RS 45, 88

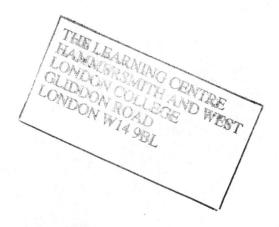

THE LEARNING CENTRE
HAMMERSMITH AND WEST
LONDON COLLEGE
GLIDDON ROAD
LONDON W14 9BL

Lightning Source UK Ltd.
Milton Keynes UK
UKOW03f1105020214

225717UK00001B/57/P

9 780719 091285